Scaphoid Fractures

Edited by
Alexander Y. Shin, MD
Professor and Consultant of Orthopedic
Surgery
Department of Orthopedic Surgery,
Division of Hand Surgery
Mayo Clinic
Rochester, Minnesota

Series Editor
Peter C. Amadio, MD
Mayo Clinic
Rochester, Minnesota

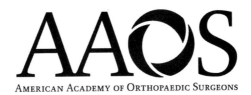

AAOS
American Academy of Orthopaedic Surgeons

Published by the
American Academy of Orthopaedic Surgeons
6300 North River Road
Rosemont, IL 60018
1-800-626-6726

The material presented in *Scaphoid Fractures* has been made available by the American Academy of Orthopaedic Surgeons for educational purposes only. This material is not intended to present the only, or necessarily best, methods or procedures for the medical situations discussed, but rather is intended to represent an approach, view, statement, or opinion of the author(s) or producer(s), which may be helpful to others who face similar situations.

Some drugs or medical devices demonstrated in Academy courses or described in Academy print or electronic publications have not been cleared by the Food and Drug Administration (FDA) or have been cleared for specific uses only. The FDA has stated that it is the responsibility of the physician to determine the FDA clearance status of each drug or device he or she wishes to use in clinical practice.

Furthermore, any statements about commercial products are solely the opinion(s) of the author(s) and do not represent an Academy endorsement or evaluation of these products. These statements may not be used in advertising or for any commercial purpose.

First Edition
Copyright © 2007 by the
American Academy of Orthopaedic Surgeons

ISBN 10: 0-89203-451-3
ISBN 13: 978-0-89203-451-2

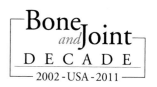

CONTRIBUTORS

Kimberly K. Amrami, MD
Assistant Professor of Radiology
Department of Radiology
Mayo Clinic
Rochester, Minnesota

Richard A. Berger, MD, PhD
Associate Dean
Department of Orthopedic Surgery, Division of
  Hand Surgery
Mayo School of Continuing Medical Education
Professor and Consultant, Orthopedic Surgery
  and Anatomy
Mayo Clinic
Rochester, Minnesota

Allen T. Bishop, MD
Professor of Orthopedic Surgery
Department of Orthopedic Surgery,
  Division of Hand Surgery
Mayo Clinic College of Medicine
Rochester, Minnesota

William P. Cooney, MD
Emeritus Consultant
Department of Orthopedic Surgery,
  Division of Hand Surgery
Mayo Clinic
Rochester, Minnesota

Bassem T. Elhassan, MD
Hand Fellow
Department of Orthopedic Surgery
Mayo Clinic
Rochester, Minnesota

Scott H. Kozin, MD
Associate Professor
Department of Orthopaedics
Temple University
Upper Extremity Surgeon
Shriners Hospital for Children
Philadelphia, Pennsylvania

Steven L. Moran, MD
Associate Professor of Orthopedic Surgery and
  Plastic Surgery
Division of Hand and Microvascular Surgery
Mayo Clinic
Rochester, Minnesota

Peter M. Murray, MD
Associate Professor
Director for Education
Department of Orthopaedic Surgery
Mayo Clinic
Jacksonville, Florida

Marco Rizzo, MD
Assistant Professor
Department of Orthopedic Surgery
Mayo Clinic
Rochester, Minnesota

Alexander Y. Shin, MD
Professor and Consultant of Orthopedic
  Surgery
Department of Orthopedic Surgery,
  Division of Hand Surgery
Mayo Clinic
Rochester, Minnesota

CONTENTS

PREFACE

The treatment of scaphoid fractures has evolved significantly over the past century. One of the earlier reports of the diagnosis and treatment of scaphoid fractures comes from 1911 in which MacLennan reported: "Fracture of the scaphoid has hitherto been regarded as a rare accident, but it is on the contrary, comparatively common. It is, however, often undetected, and a diagnosis of sprained wrist is accepted as explaining the symptoms. Even when a skiagram is taken, the fracture may escape notice, as the scrutiny of the plate is concentrated upon the lower end of the radius."[1] In describing the treatment, MacLennan stated that "Operative treatment may be divided into attempts to wire the fragments, to remove the upper and more displaced one, or to remove both fragments. The wiring of the fragments is seldom practicable; it takes time and really causes considerable interference with surrounding structures. Excision of one or both fragments is rapidly performed without damaging the neighbouring parts, and gives the best results."[1]

This attitude regarding the treatment of scaphoid fractures persisted for nearly 50 years until Fisk in his Hunterian lectures described the association of carpal deformity secondary to scaphoid fracture nonunions[2]. Further understanding of the importance of the scaphoid in carpal kinematics and traumatic wrist instability was introduced by Linscheid, Dobyns and Beabout in 1972[3].

Over the past several decades, advances in radiographic imaging, clearer knowledge of the anatomy of the scaphoid, understanding of the carpal kinematics, attempts at ascertaining the natural history of the scaphoid nonunion as well as innovation in treatment of scaphoid fractures and nonunion has significantly benefited our patients.

The treatment of scaphoid fractures can be simple or complex, mundane or exhilarating, and satisfying or frustrating. In this monograph, all aspects of scaphoid fractures and nonunions are explored: the anatomy, radiology, treatment of acute and chronic injuries, pediatric injuries, scaphoid fractures associated with osteonecrosis of the proximal pole and with associated perilunar instabilities, and salvage options for nonsalvagable scaphoid nonunions.

I would like to express my appreciation and sincere thanks to the authors for their outstanding contributions and to the American Academy of Orthopaedic Surgeons for their support of this publication. It has been a pleasure to work with such talented surgeons who are leaders in this field. This monograph will prove to be an excellent reference for the treatment of scaphoid fractures and nonunions.

Alexander Y. Shin, MD
Professor and Consultant of Orthopedic
 Surgery
Department of Orthopedic Surgery,
 Division of Hand Surgery
Mayo Clinic
Rochester, Minnesota

1. MacLennan A: The treatment of fracture of the carpal scaphoid and the indications for operation. *British Medical Journal* 1911;1089.
2. Fisk GR: Carpal instability and the fractured scaphoid. *Ann R Coll Surg Engl* 1970;46:63.
3. Linscheid RL, Dobyns JH, Beabout JW, et al: Traumatic instability of the wrist: Diagnosis, classification, and pathomechanics. *J Bone Joint Surg Am* 1972;54:1612.

CHAPTER 1

SCAPHOID FRACTURES AND NONUNIONS

MARCO RIZZO, MD
ALEXANDER Y. SHIN, MD

Our understanding and treatment of scaphoid fractures has widely expanded over the last 50 years. Early recommendations for unhealed fractures included benign neglect and excision.[1] Unfortunately, it became readily apparent that the consequences of scaphoid malunion or nonunion frequently correlated with a poor functional outcome and osteoarthritis. With a better understanding of the anatomy, diagnosis, and treatment, improved healing and patient outcomes can be achieved. Both the diagnosis and treatment of acute scaphoid fractures have improved tremendously over the past 20 years, resulting in increased awareness, improved diagnostic modalities, advances in surgical techniques and implants, and improved treatment regimens. Despite these advances, however, treatment of scaphoid fractures remains a difficult problem.

INCIDENCE

The exact incidence of scaphoid fractures has been somewhat difficult to quantify,[2-8] particularly because many of these injuries are frequently undiagnosed. One estimate is that scaphoid fractures represent 60% to 70% of all carpal bone fractures and 2% to 7% of all fractures seen in the emergency department.[9,10] One study estimates that the average incidence is 35 scaphoid fractures per year for a hospital serving a quarter of a million people.[11]

Scaphoid fractures typically occur in active, energetic adolescents and young adults, with an incidence two to four times higher in men than in women.[2,3,8,10] In an epidemiologic study of scaphoid fractures evaluated over a 3-year period in the Norwegian population, Hove[12] noted a 2% incidence of scaphoid fractures among all bone injuries. Scaphoid fractures represented 11% of all hand and 60% of all carpal bone fractures. Men outnumbered women by 4:1 ratio, with 20- to 30-year-old adults most commonly affected. The overall annual incidence was 4.3 in 10,000 people.

Fortunately, most scaphoid fractures treated nonsurgically heal without consequence, with the incidence of nonunion reported to be between 5% and 15%.[8,13,14] If untreated, scaphoid fractures progress to carpal collapse followed by eventual radiocarpal then midcarpal osteoarthritic changes.[15,16]

MECHANISM OF INJURY

The fracture most commonly occurs as a result of a violent dorsiflexion of the wrist from a fall or protective maneuver against the outstretched arm.[17] Frykman[18] showed that cadaver specimens subjected to forceful extension were more likely to demonstrate scaphoid fractures when the wrist was hyperextended and radially deviated, whereas distal radius fractures were more likely to be produced at lesser angles of extension and smaller loads. Weber and Chao[19] were able to produce scaphoid fractures in 10 cadaver arms by applying a load between 209 and 436 kg of force when the wrist was extended past 95° and radially deviated more than 10°. They showed that during this loading condition, virtually all of the force across the wrist was transmitted through the scaphoid. At the same time, the component of the radiocarpal capsule (radial collateral ligament) extending from the radial styloid to the scaphoid tuberosity was relaxed by the radial deviation. This failed to relieve the tensile stresses in the palmar cortex of the scaphoid in this configuration. Its proximal pole was locked tightly into the scaphoid fossa of the radius by the radiolunate and radiocapitate ligaments stretched across the scaphoid waist, and its distal pole was angulated dorsally beyond its normal limit of motion. As a result, the scaphoid fractured in tension beginning at the palmar cortex, identical with classic beam-loading experiments of basic mechanics.

In this model, the tensile stresses on the deflected side of the beam become smaller as they approach the side of the beam under compression. From this null point, the internal stresses are then compressive and, if material failure occurs, the fracture seam extends in a Y-like fashion along the shear stress lines at the theoretical ideal 45° angles. This accounts for the dorsal comminution seen, for instance, in distal radius fractures. Dorsal or dorsoradial comminution in scaphoid fractures is, however, much less common. The reason for this may lie in the give afforded by the midcarpal joint. This allows the null point of the tensile stresses to approach or lie beyond the dorsal cortex of the scaphoid. Because tensile fractures usually are transverse, this may help to explain why fractures of the scaphoid waist are generally rather clean breaks. There are, of course, exceptions to this observation, especially in transscaphoid perilunate dislocations.[20-24] Stress fractures of the scaphoid also have been identified.[25] Other mechanisms for scaphoid fractures have included the axially loading (puncher's) fracture,[26] coronal scaphoid fractures,[27] and avulsions of the distal pole of the scaphoid.[22]

DIAGNOSIS

Physical Examination

Most patients with acute scaphoid fractures present with pain and swelling in the wrist. In higher energy injuries, there may be concomitant injuries, which can mask the scaphoid injury. Another common presentation is persistent pain after a fall onto an outstretched hand that has not improved despite splinting and anti-inflamma-tory medications. These patients often no longer have swelling but can have limited motion and weakness of the affected wrist.

Snuffbox tenderness is a classic presenting finding on examination.[28] In fact, we believe that snuffbox tenderness in a patient with antecedent trauma is a conclusive sign of scaphoid fracture until proved otherwise. However, snuffbox tenderness may be absent in the presence of a fracture, especially in the subacute or chronic setting. The most accurate examination finding in a swollen wrist is the scaphoid compression test, in which an axial load from the first ray is placed on the scaphoid.[29,30] Other examination findings include pain over the scaphoid tubercle,[31] pain with resisted pronation,[32] and pain with attempted scaphoid shift test. Some of these findings are typically associated with scapholunate ligament injury but can exist in the setting of acute fracture. Parvizi and associates[33] attempted to verify the accuracy of physical examination findings and found sensitivity of snuffbox and tubercle tenderness to be 100%, but specificity was only 9% for snuffbox tenderness and 30% for scaphoid tubercle. The most specific examination finding was painful thumb motion at 48%. When they combined these three tests, the specificity increased to 74%. In another study,[34] anatomic snuffbox tenderness alone was 100% sensitive, 76% specific, and carried a 92% positive predictive value for fracture.

In some patients, the diagnosis will be an acute on chronic situation. A recent trauma presents as an acute injury but may in fact be an exacerbation of an older fracture.[35,36] It is important to discern the timing of the initial fracture because treatment options may differ. A thorough history, including previous falls or injuries of the wrist, and radiographic evaluation are helpful.

Radiographic Evaluation

Plain radiographs should be ordered for all patients with suspected scaphoid fractures. Between three and six views of the wrist have been recommended,[34,37-39] specifically AP and/or posteroanterior (PA), lateral, oblique and scaphoid views (**Figure 1**). The scaphoid view is a special PA of the wrist in ulnar deviation, pronated obliquely at 45° and ulnarly elevated at 45°.[40] Mehta and Brautigan[34] advocate six views: the four standard views, a 25° pronated, and a 25° supinated view. They found that with the six-view series, no scaphoid

FIGURE 1

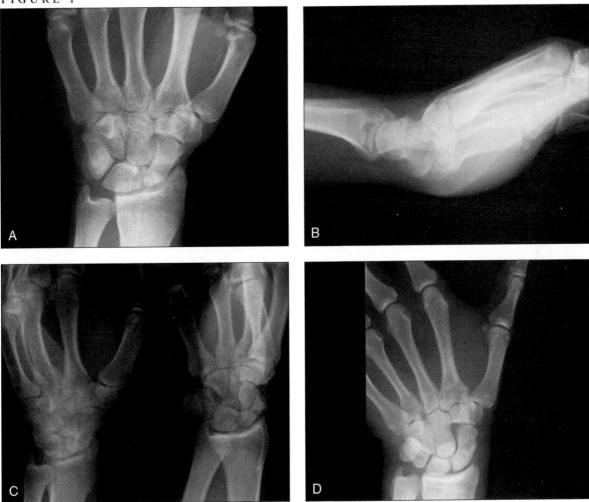

Four radiographic views of the wrist typically obtained in patients with suspected scaphoid fractures: PA **(A)**, lateral **(B)**, and two oblique images **(C)**. **D,** The scaphoid view allows for a view of the scaphoid in its true coronal plane. The wrist is extended and ulnarly deviated and the x-ray beam is oriented in line with the thumb.

fractures were missed in a consecutive series of 90 patients, whereas with just the four-view series, 11 were missed. Roolker and associates[41] noted improved diagnostic accuracy of scaphoid fractures with the use of a carpal box radiograph in which elongated and magnified views of the scaphoid are obtained with the film cassette angled (approximately 50°) below the hand.

It is not uncommon for a patient to have normal radiographs and persistent pain. Traditional management for these patients includes immobilization in a thumb spica cast and follow-up radiographs in 2 weeks. Typi-cally, later radiographs demonstrate a sclerotic line, if it is in fact a scaphoid fracture. However, diagnostic modalities such as CT,[42-45] technetium Tc 99m bone scan,[46-52] ultrasound,[53-56] and MRI[57-62] have all demonstrated efficacy in diagnosing occult scaphoid fractures.

Technetium Tc 99m bone scans have demonstrated 100% sensitivity in diagnosing acute scaphoid fractures[46] (**Figure 2**). Most fractures have increased uptake at the injury site within 24 to 48 hours, making a bone scan obtained after that period of time effective, with

FIGURE 2

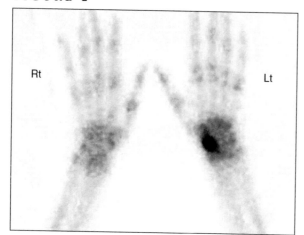

Bone scan of a patient with a scaphoid fracture. The hot spot corresponds to the fracture site.

FIGURE 3

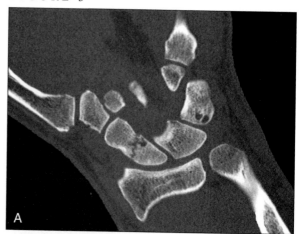

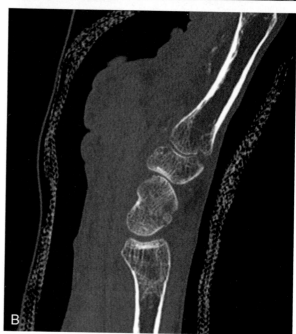

A, Coronal CT scan of a minimally displaced scaphoid fracture. B, In the sagittal plane, the scan should be performed in the longitudinal axis of the scaphoid.

improved accuracy as time from injury increases.[63] Bone scan also is useful in diagnosing concomitant or other injuries.[48] A disadvantage of bone scans is that although very sensitive, they lack specificity for scaphoid fractures. A 15% false-positive rate has been reported.[64] Patients with preexisting conditions such as arthrosis, cysts, or synovitis can confound the accuracy of diagnosis. A second shortcoming of three-phase bone scans are that they provide little information regarding specific fracture location.

Ultrasound also has demonstrated efficacy in diagnosing occult scaphoid fractures. It is generally less expensive than modalities such as MRI and it lacks the ionizing radiation of CT. Hauger and associates[56] reported greater success in cases with cortical disruption of the scaphoid and the presence of hemarthrosis. Among 54 patients studied, they experienced only one false-positive result. Finkenberg and associates[53] reported on intrasound vibration for diagnosis of scaphoid fractures with favorable sensitivity and specificity. However, subsequent studies have failed to repeat their success.[65,66] Unfortunately, this variability underscores the fact that success with ultrasound is institution and technician dependent. Another shortcoming is that ultrasound offers little or no information regarding the structural integrity of the scaphoid or associated injuries.

In suspected scaphoid fractures, CT is commonly used for assessment, as well as for providing specific bony

detail to known fractures. Scanning should be oriented to the longitudinal axis of the scaphoid[42] (**Figure 3**) so that the presence of a humpback deformity can be identified in existing fractures or nonunions. Parameters such as interscaphoid angle and height-to-length ratios are calculated from this view and help with surgical decision making and planning. The interscaphoid angle is

FIGURE 4

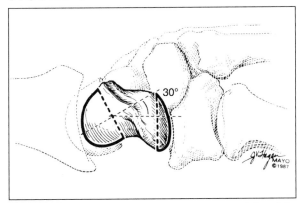

The interscaphoid angle is measured based on the lateral view of the bone. It helps to determine the presence of collapse or humpback deformity. The normal angle is 35°. (Reproduced with permission from Amadio PC, Berquist TH, Smith DK, et al: Scaphoid malunion. *J Hand Surg Am* 1989;14:680.)

FIGURE 5

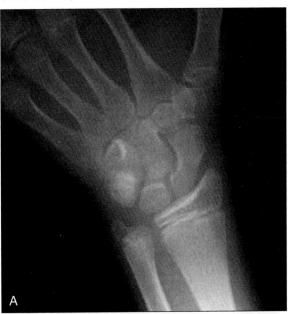

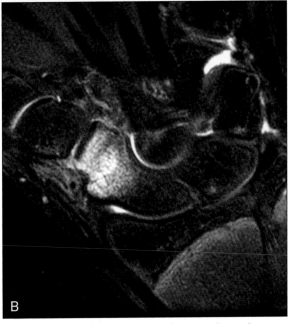

A, PA view of a patient with a scaphoid fracture and normal-appearing radiograph. **B,** MRI scan demonstrates edema across the scaphoid, consistent with an occult fracture.

determined by drawing separate perpendicular lines from the proximal and distal poles and calculating the angle of intersection.[67] A normal angle is approximately 35° and increases in the presence of a humpback deformity or malunion. Height-to-length ratio is measured on the same views and is normally less than 0.6542 (**Figure 4**). Thin, 1-mm cuts are recommended to maximize the detail and allow for improved reconstructed three-dimensional images.[45] CT is also advantageous in identifying additional bony injuries. Although extremely useful in evaluating the architecture of the scaphoid, one study found that CT had 14% false-negative rates in diagnosing occult fractures.[68]

The most reliable means of identifying occult scaphoid fractures is MRI.[52] It has become the modality of choice in our institution for ruling out (or confirming) a scaphoid fracture (**Figures 5 and 6**)

CLASSIFICATION

A useful classification scheme helps to plan treatment and predict outcomes. Numerous systems for acute scaphoid fractures have been reported.[25,28,37,69-74] Classification can be based on two parameters: anatomic location and fracture stability. Russe[74] reported a classification system based on the obliquity of the fracture line (**Figure 7**). Vertical fractures were inherently more unstable, whereas horizontal oblique and transverse frac-

tures were more stable. McLaughlin and Parkes[25] described a classification based on extent of fracture and degree of displacement. Type A fractures were incom-

FIGURE 6

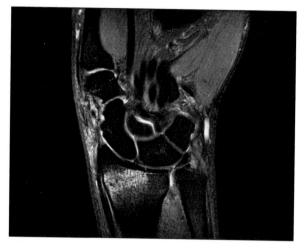

MRI scan of a patient with suspected scaphoid fracture and normal plain radiographs shows an associated nondisplaced fracture of the radial styloid.

FIGURE 7

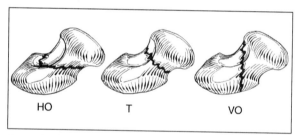

HO   T   VO

Russe classification system for scaphoid fractures. HO = Horizontal oblique; VO = vertical oblique; T = transverse. (Reproduced with permission from Linscheid RL, Weber ER: Scaphoid fractures and nonunions, in Cooney WP (ed): *The Wrist.* St Louis, MO, Mosby, 1998, p 394.)

FIGURE 8

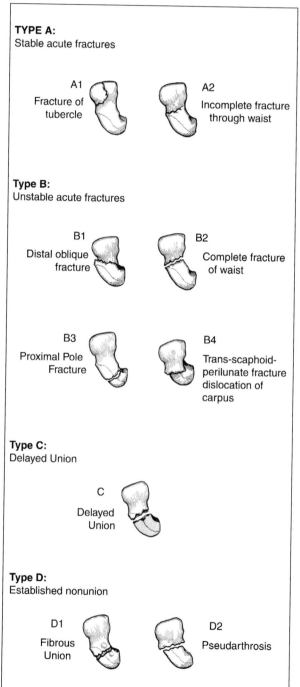

TYPE A:
Stable acute fractures

A1
Fracture of tubercle

A2
Incomplete fracture through waist

Type B:
Unstable acute fractures

B1
Distal oblique fracture

B2
Complete fracture of waist

B3
Proximal Pole Fracture

B4
Trans-scaphoid-perilunate fracture dislocation of carpus

Type C:
Delayed Union

C
Delayed Union

Type D:
Established nonunion

D1
Fibrous Union

D2
Pseudarthrosis

Herbert classification of scaphoid fractures. (Reproduced with permission from Linscheid RL, Weber ER: Scaphoid fractures and nonunions, in Cooney WP (ed): *The Wrist.* St Louis, MO, Mosby, 1998, p 394.)

plete, type B were complete without displacement, and type C were displaced. They went on to recommend treatment based on type of fracture: splinting (for type A), cast immobilization or surgery (for type B), and surgery (for type C). Weber's classification also included three groups: (1) nondisplaced, (2) angulated, and (3) displaced.[72] Healing rates progressively decreased based on the fracture type. Herbert and Fisher[73] described a more elaborate system (**Figure 8**). This classification attempts to guide surgical treatment by again attempting to target the more unstable fractures. Stable (type

FIGURE 9

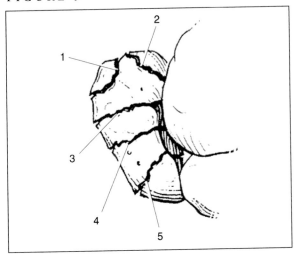

Mayo classification for scaphoid fractures based on location. Types 1 and 2 are distal pole fractures. Type 3 is a distal third fracture, type 4 is a midwaist fracture, and type 5 is a proximal pole fracture. (Reproduced with permission from Linscheid RL, Weber ER: Scaphoid fractures and nonunions, in Cooney WP (ed): *The Wrist.* St Louis, MO, Mosby, 1998, p 394.)

FIGURE 10

Location	Number of fractures	% Union
Distal 1/3	2	100
Middle 1/3	56	80
Proximal 1/3	32	64

Displacement	Number of fractures	% Union
Stable	48	85
Unstable	42	65

Incidence of fracture location of the scaphoid and associated healing rates. (Reproduced with permission from Cooney WP III: Scaphoid fractures: Current treatments and techniques. *Instr Course Lect* 2003;52:201.)

A) fractures include tubercle and incomplete nondisplaced waist fractures. Unstable (type B) fractures are distal oblique, complete waist fractures, proximal pole fractures, and fractures associated with perilunate dislocations. Types C and D related to chronic fractures and nonunions. Type C fractures are delayed unions, whereas type D are chronic or established nonunions with either a fibrous union (type D1) or pseudarthrosis (type D2). Because of difficulties with predicting fracture healing with some of these radiographic systems,[75] modifications have been proposed using better imaging techniques. Karle and associates[43] recently introduced a CT-based classification to enhance the predictive stability of the Herbert classification. The authors recommend CT to justify nonsurgical treatment because they strongly feel that plain radiographs underestimate the degree of displacement or comminution. The Mayo classification[37] based on location identifies five fracture sites: (1) distal tubercle, (2) distal intra-articular, (3) distal third, (4) waist, and (5) proximal pole (**Figure 9**). In addition to location, the Mayo classification system defines acute fractures based on their stability. Stable fractures have less than 1 mm displacement, normal carpal alignment, and interscaphoid angulation. Fracture healing rates based on both location and stability are detailed in **Figure 10**.[37]

NATURAL HISTORY OF SCAPHOID NONUNIONS

The propensity of the scaphoid to proceed to nonunion and, as is now recognized, to malunion is attributable to several features.[67,76] Gilford and associates[77] recognized the inherent tendency of the midcarpal joint to undergo a collapse with scaphoid nonunion, which was described as a "stop-link" mechanism. Fisk[5,76] elaborated on this in his Hunterian lecture in 1968, referring to this as the "concertina effect" (**Figure 11**).[77] A generic term for traumatic carpal instability, in which the proximal carpal row as represented by the lunate might assume either a flexed or an extended posture when destabilized, was introduced later. The terms volar intercalated segment instability (VISI) and dorsal intercalated segment instability (DISI) were introduced to signify these unstable postures.[78] That this instability was the cause rather than the result of malunion and nonunion slowly became apparent.

The scaphoid lies obliquely across the midcarpal joint

FIGURE 11

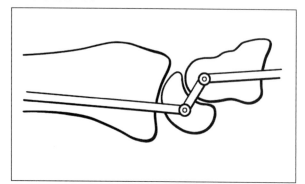

The stop-link mechanism associated with scaphoid fractures. The carpus collapses, leading to extension of the lunate and subsequent increase in the lunocapitate angle. (Copyright Mayo Foundation, 2007.)

FIGURE 12

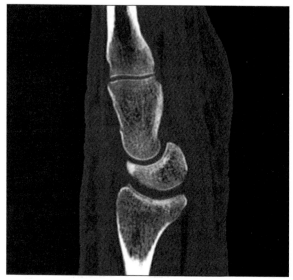

Sagittal view of the lunate in patient with a scaphoid fracture and collapse. Note the extension of the lunate and DISI deformity.

FIGURE 13

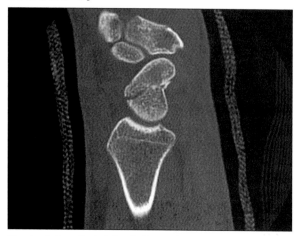

The classic humpback deformity frequently associated with displaced and/or comminuted scaphoid fractures. The deforming forces force the distal pole into flexion.

on its radial aspect at approximately 45°, where it acts to stabilize the highly unstable midcarpal joint.[78] Normally, compression of the scaphoid between the radius and trapezium acts to flex the scaphoid and, through the scapholunate ligament complex, the lunate as well. The counterbalance to this tendency is the normal action of the triquetrum to extend. Both of these bones, through their ligamentous attachment to the lunate, try to influence its angulation, but in opposite directions.[79] If the balancing act fails, the lunate angulates under the more influential neighboring bone. A fracture disrupts

the scaphoid influence and allows the lunate to assume an extended position. This DISI may not be immediately apparent, but during protracted inherent compressive forces, the angle between the capitate and lunate increases insidiously (**Figure 12**). The proximal pole of the scaphoid is also extended through the scapholunate ligament complex. This tends to gap open the fracture site, markedly decreasing the coaptive surfaces through which bony healing would occur. Erosion of the palmar cortices through repetitive micromotion shortens the palmar length. If it should heal in this position, it gives rise to the so-called humpback deformity (**Figure 13**).[76,78,80]

The distal pole also tends to translate dorsally on the proximal segment of the scaphoid under the influence of the capitate that has "ridden up" in the lunate concavity. Angulation and displacement are also evident in the coronal plane, usually as an apex radial angulation, and in the transverse plane, as pronation of the distal fragment. Three-dimensional reconstruction makes these changes much more evident.[81] The nonunion problem is then likely to be a biomechanical one and is compounded by deficient vascularity to varying degrees as well as difficulty in achieving adequate immobilization.[82] Kinematics of the wrist are altered progressively by the intracarpal distortions.[38,15,16,83]

Clinically, the natural history of nonunion leads to a predictable pattern of arthritis referred to as scaphoid nonunion advanced collapse wrist.[67,84] With improved diagnostic modalities and increased awareness, the incidence of premature carpal collapse and arthritis is higher than previously appreciated.[85] Although difficult to determine for certain, many authors agree that scaphoid nonunion leads to osteoarthritis within 10 years.[86-88] There appears to be a clear relationship between the loss of its blood supply, displaced fractures, proximal fractures, inadequate/inappropriate treatment and comminution, and the development of scaphoid nonunion.[3] Like most difficult problems, scaphoid nonunions are rarely painful in the early stages.[85,86,88] And like most difficult problems, there appears to be a negative relationship between duration of nonunion and success of treatment.[84] This information is somewhat incomplete because of the nature of scaphoid nonunions. It often is difficult to determine the duration of a nonunion and thus it is difficult to confirm precisely the natural history. Much like scapholunate advanced collapse wrists, the scaphoid nonunion advance collapse may have a silent population who never seek attention. Despite this possibility, prevention remains the best treatment.

CONCLUSION

The scaphoid is a key element in the carpal functions of the wrist. It is quite susceptible to injury and fracture and requires prompt diagnosis and definitive treatment. Early diagnosis and appropriate treatment usually results in fracture union and avoids fracture nonunion. A thorough understanding of the anatomy, pathomechanics of the wrist, and treatment options is necessary in planning the optimal course of action for patients with scaphoid nonunion.

REFERENCES

1. Boyd H: Fractures, in Speed J, Smith H (eds): *Campbell's Operative Orthopaedics*, ed 2. St. Louis, CV Mosby, vol 1, 1949, p 527.

2. Osterman AL, Mikulics M: Scaphoid nonunion. *Hand Clin* 1988;4:437-455.

3. Trumble E, Salas P, Barthel T, Robert KQ III: Management of scaphoid nonunions. *J Am Acad Orthop Surg* 2003;11:380-391.

4. Borgeskov S, Christiansen B, Kjaer A, Balslev I: Fractures of the carpal bones. *Acta Orthop Scand* 1966;37:276-287.

5. Fisk GR: Carpal instability and the fractured scaphoid. *Ann R Coll Surg Engl* 1970;46:63-76.

6. London PS: The broken scaphoid bone: The case against pessimism. *J Bone Joint Surg Br* 1961;43:237-244.

7. Kozin SH: Incidence, mechanism, and natural history of scaphoid fractures. *Hand Clin* 2001;17:515-524.

8. Kuschner SH, Lane CS, Brien WW, Gellman H: Scaphoid fractures and scaphoid nonunion: Diagnosis and treatment. *Orthop Rev* 1994;23:861-871.

9. Pillai A, Jain M: Management of clinical fractures of the scaphoid: Results of an audit and literature review. *Eur J Emerg Med* 2005;12:47-51.

10. Grover R: Clinical assessment of scaphoid injuries and the detection of fractures. *J Hand Surg Br* 1996;21:341-343.

11. Barton NJ: Twenty questions about scaphoid fractures. *J Hand Surg Br* 1992;17:289-310.

12. Hove LM: Epidemiology of scaphoid fractures in Bergen, Norway. *Scand J Plast Reconstr Surg Hand Surg* 1999;33:423-426.

13. Gellman H, Caputo RJ, Carter V, Aboulafia A, McKay M: Comparison of short and long thumb-spica casts for non-displaced fractures of the carpal scaphoid [see comments]. *J Bone Joint Surg Am* 1989;71:354-357.

14. Dias JJ, Taylor M, Thompson J, Brenkel IJ, Gregg PJ: Radiographic signs of union of scaphoid fractures: An analysis of interobserver agreement and reproducibility. *J Bone Joint Surg Br* 1988;70:299-301.

15. Youm Y, McMurthy RY, Flatt AE, Gillespie TE: Kinematics of the wrist: I. An experimental study of radial-ulnar deviation and flexion-extension. *J Bone Joint Surg Am* 1978;60:423-431.

16. Burgess RC: The effect of a simulated scaphoid malunion on wrist motion. *J Hand Surg Am* 1987;12:774-776.

17. Rongieres M, Mansat M, Bonnevialle P, Darmana R, Railhac JJ: [Pathomechanics of fractures of the scaphoid]. *Rev Chir Orthop Reparatrice Appar Mot* 1988;74:689-692.

18. Frykman GK: Fracture of the distal radius including sequelae: Shoulder-hand-finger syndrome, disturbance in the distal radio ulnar joint and impairment of nerve

function. A clinical and experimental study. *Acta Orthop Scand* 1967(Suppl);108:3.

19. Weber ER, Chao EYS: An experimental approach to the mechanism of scaphoid waist fractures. *J Hand Surg* 1978;3:142-148.

20. Herzberg G: [Fractures and pseudarthroses of the carpal scaphoid: Results concerning type II, III and IV fractures combined with ligament lesions (luxation or peri-lunate trans-scaphoid subluxation)]. *Rev Chir Orthop Reparatrice Appar Mot* 1988;74:711-713.

21. Herzberg G, Allieu Y: [Fractures and pseudarthroses of the carpal scaphoid. Combined bone and ligament lesions in fresh fractures: An anatomo-radiologic analysis]. *Rev Chir Orthop Reparatrice Appar Mot* 1988;74:695-697.

22. Compson JP, Waterman JK, Spencer JD: Dorsal avulsion fractures of the scaphoid: Diagnostic implications and applied anatomy. *J Hand Surg Br* 1993;18:58-61.

23. Green DP, O'Brien ET: Open reduction of carpal dislocations: Indications and operative techniques. *J Hand Surg Am* 1978;3:250-265.

24. Eglseder WA, Ross G: Transscaphoid palmar lunate dislocation with scapholunate dissociation. *Mil Med* 1992;157:382-385.

25. McLaughlin HL, Parkes JC: Fracture of the carpal navicular (scaphoid) bone: Gradations in therapy based upon pathology. *J Trauma* 1969;9:311-319.

26. Horii E, Nakamura R, Watanabe K, Tsunoda K: Scaphoid fracture as a "puncher's fracture." *J Orthop Trauma* 1994;8:107-110.

27. Shin AY, Horton T, Bishop AT: Acute coronal plane scaphoid fracture and scapholunate dissociation from an axial load: A case report. *J Hand Surg Am* 2005;30:366-372.

28. Cooney WP, Dobyns JH, Linscheid RL: Fractures of the scaphoid: A rational approach to management. *Clin Orthop* 1980;149:90-97.

29. Chen SC: The scaphoid compression test. *J Hand Surg Br* 1989;14:323-325.

30. Grover R: Clinical assessment of scaphoid injuries and the detection of fractures. *J Hand Surg Br* 1996;21:341-343.

31. Freeland P: Scaphoid tubercle tenderness: A better indictor of scaphoid fractures? *Arch Emerg Med* 1989;6:46-50.

32. Verdan C, Narakas A: Fractures and pseudarthrosis of the scaphoid. *Surg Clin North Am* 1968;48:1083-1095.

33. Parvizi J, Wayman J, Kelly P, Moran CG: Combining the clinical signs improves diagnosis of scaphoid fractures: A prospective study with follow-up. *J Hand Surg Br* 1998;23:324-327.

34. Mehta M, Brautigan MW: Fracture of the carpal navicular: Efficacy of clinical findings and improved diagnosis with six-view radiography. *Ann Emerg Med* 1990;19:255-257.

35. Tiel-van Buul MM, Roolker W, Broekhuizen AH, Van Beek EJ: The diagnostic management of suspected scaphoid fracture. *Injury* 1997;28:1-8.

36. Dias JJ, Thompson J, Barton NJ, Gregg PJ: Suspected scaphoid fractures. The value of radiographs. *J Bone Joint Surg Br* 1990;72:98-101.

37. Cooney WP III: Scaphoid fractures: Current treatments and techniques. *Instr Course Lect* 2003;52:197-208.

38. Leslie IJ, Dickson RA: The fractured carpal scaphoid: Natural history and factors influencing outcome. *J Bone Joint Surg Br* 1981;63:225.

39. Rettig AC: Management of acute scaphoid fractures. *Hand Clin* 2000;16:381-395.

40. Jupiter JB, Shin AY, Trumble TE, Fernandez DL: Traumatic and reconstructive problems of the scaphoid. *Instr Course Lect* 2001;50:105-122.

41. Roolker W, Tiel-van Buul MM, Bossuyt PM, et al: Carpal box radiography in suspected scaphoid fracture. *J Bone Joint Surg Br* 1996;78:535-539.

42. Sanders WE: Evaluation of the humpback scaphoid by computed tomography in the longitudinal axial plane of the scaphoid. *J Hand Surg Am* 1988;13:182-187.

43. Karle B, Mayer B, Kitzinger HB, Frohner S, Schmitt R, Krimmer H: [Scaphoid fractures: Operative or conservative treatment? A CT-based classification]. *Handchir Mikrochir Plast Chir* 2005;37:260-266.

44. Bain GI, Bennett JD, Richards RS, Slethaug GP, Roth JH: Longitudinal computer tomography of the scaphoid: A new technique. *Skeletal Radiol* 1995;24:271-273.

45. Nakamura R, Imaeda T, Horii E, Miura T, Hayakawa N: Analysis of scaphoid fracture displacement by three-dimensional computed tomography. *J Hand Surg Am* 1991;16:485-492.

46. Ganel A, Engel J, Oster Z, Farine I: Bone scanning in the assessment of fractures of the scaphoid. *J Hand Surg Am* 1979;4:540-543.

47. Brown JN: The suspected scaphoid fracture and isotope bone imaging. *Injury* 1995;26:479-482.

48. Murphy D, Eisenhauer M: The utility of a bone scan in the diagnosis of clinical scaphoid fracture. *J Emerg Med* 1994;12:709-712.

49. Tiel-van Buul MM, Roolker W, Verbeeten BW, Broekhuizen AH: Magnetic resonance imaging versus bone scintigraphy in suspected scaphoid fracture. *Eur J Nucl Med* 1996;23:971-975.

50. Waizenegger M, Wastie ML, Barton NJ, Davis TR: Scintigraphy in the evaluation of the "clinical" scaphoid fracture. *J Biomech Br* 1994;19:750-753.

51. Wilson AW, Kurer MH, Peggington JL, Grant DS, Kirk CC: Bone scintigraphy in the management of x-ray negative potential scaphoid fractures. *Arch Emerg Med* 1986;3:235-242.

52. Fowler C, Sullivan B, Williams LA, McCarthy G, Savage R, Palmer A: A comparison of bone scintigraphy and MRI in the early diagnosis of the occult scaphoid waist fracture. *Skeletal Radiol* 1998;27:683-687.

53. Finkenberg JG, Hoffer E, Kelly C, Zinar DM: Diagnosis of occult scaphoid fractures by intrasound vibration. *J Hand Surg Am* 1993;18:4-7.

54. Senall JA, Failla JM, Bouffard JA, van Holsbeeck M: Ultrasound for the early diagnosis of clinically suspected scaphoid fracture. *J Hand Surg Am* 2004;29:400-405.

55. Christiansen TG, Rude C, Lauridsen KK, Christensen OM: Diagnostic value of ultrasound in scaphoid fractures. *Injury* 1991;22:397-399.

56. Hauger O, Bonnefoy O, Moinard M, Bersani D, Diard F: Occult fractures of the waist of the scaphoid: Early diagnosis by high-spatial-resolution sonography. *AJR Am J Roentgenol* 2002;178:1239-1245.

57. Raby N: Magnetic resonance imaging of suspected scaphoid fractures using a low field dedicated extremity MR system. *Clin Radiol* 2001;56:316-320.

58. Breitenseher MJ, Metz VM, Gilula LA, et al: Radiographically occult scaphoid fractures: Value of MR imaging in detection. *Radiology* 1997;203:245-250.

59. Gaebler C, Kukla C, Breitenseher M, Trattnig S, Mittlboeck M, Vecsei V: Magnetic resonance imaging of occult scaphoid fractures. *J Trauma* 1996;41:73-76.

60. Hunter JC, Escobedo EM, Wilson AJ, Hanel DP, Zink-Brody GC, Mann FA: MR imaging of clinically suspected scaphoid fractures. *AJR Am J Roentgenol* 1997;168:1287-1293.

61. Imaeda T, Nakamura R, Miura T, Makino N: Magnetic resonance imaging in scaphoid fractures. *J Hand Surg Br* 1992;17:20-27.

62. Moller JM, Larsen L, Bovin J, et al: MRI diagnosis of fracture of the scaphoid bone: Impact of a new practice where the images are read by radiographers. *Acad Radiol* 2004;11:724-728.

63. Tiel-van Buul MM, van Beek EJ, Borm JJ, Gubler FM, Broekhuizen AH, van Royen EA: The value of radiographs and bone scintigraphy in suspected scaphoid fracture, a statistical analysis. *J Hand Surg Br* 1993;18:403-406.

64. Murphy DG, Eisenhauer MA, Powe J, Pavlofsky W: Can a day 4 bone scan accurately determine the presence or absence of scaphoid fracture? *Ann Emerg Med* 1995;26:434-438.

65. Roolker L, Tiel-van Buul MM, Broekhuizen TH: Is intrasound vibration useful in the diagnosis of occult scaphoid fractures? *J Hand Surg Am* 1998;23:229-232.

66. Knight P, Rothwell AG: Intrasound vibration in the early diagnosis of scaphoid fracture. *J Hand Surg Am* 1998;23:233-235.

67. Amadio PC, Berquist TH, Smith DK, Ilstrup DM, Cooney WP III, Linscheid RL: Scaphoid malunion. *J Hand Surg Am* 1989;14:679-687.

68. Tiel-van Buul MM, van Beek EJ, Dijkstra PF, Bakker AJ, Broekhuizen TH, van Royen EA: Significance of a hot spot on the bone scan after carpal injury: Evaluation by computed tomography. *Eur J Nucl Med* 1993;20:159-164.

69. Muller M, Allgower M, Willenegger H: *Manual of Internal Fixation*. Berlin, Germany, Springer-Verlag, 1970.

70. Sennwald G: *The Wrist: Anatomical and Pathophysiological Approach to Diagnosis and Treatment*. Berlin, Germany, Springer-Verlag, 1987, pp 83-98.

71. Schernberg F: [Classification of fractures of the carpal scaphoid: An anatomo-radiologic study of characteristics]. *Rev Chir Orthop Reparatrice Appar Mot* 1988;74:693-695.

72. Weber ER: Biomechanical implications of scaphoid waist fractures. *Clin Orthop* 1980;149:83-89.

73. Herbert TJ, Fisher WE: Management of the fractured scaphoid using a new bone screw. *J Bone Joint Surg Br* 1984;66:114-123.

74. Russe O: Fracture of the carpal navicular: Diagnosis, nonoperative treatment and operative treatment. *J Bone Joint Surg Am* 1960;42:759-768.

75. Desai V, Davis TRC, Barton NJ: The prognostic value and reproducibility of the radiological features of the fractured scaphoid. *J Hand Surg Br* 1999;24:586-590.

76. Linscheid RL, Dobyns J, Cooney WP III: Pathogenesis of carpal scaphoid nonunion and malunion with biomechanical analysis (abstract). *Orthop Trans* 1983;7:482.

77. Gilford WW, Bolton RH, Lambrinudi C: The mechanism of the wrist joint, with special reference to fractures of the scaphoid. *Guys Hosp Rep* 1943;92:52-59.

78. Fisk GR: Non-union of the carpal scaphoid treated by wedge grafting (abstract). *J Bone Joint Surg Br* 1984;66:277.

79. Linscheid RL, Dobyns JH, Beabout JW, Bryan RS: Traumatic instability of the wrist: Diagnosis, classification, and pathomechanics. *J Bone Joint Surg Am* 1972;54:1612-1632.

80. Berger RA: The anatomy of the scaphoid. *Hand Clin* 2001;17:525-532.

81. Dias JJ, Brenkel IJ, Finlay DB: Patterns of union in fractures of the waist of the scaphoid. *J Bone Joint Surg Br* 1989;71:307-310.

82. Belsole RJ, Hilbelink DR, Llewellyn JA, Dale M, Greene TL, Rayhack JM: Computed analyses of the pathomechanics of scaphoid waist nonunions. *J Hand Surg* 1991;16:899-906.

83. Mjoberg B: Wrist joint tamponade after scaphoid fracture: A case report. *Acta Orthop Scand* 1989;60:371.

84. Smith DK, Cooney WP III, An KN, Linscheid RL, Chao EY: The effects of simulated unstable scaphoid fractures on carpal motion. *J Hand Surg Am* 1989;14:283-291.

85. Trumble TE, Clarke T, Kreder HJ: Non-union of the scaphoid: Treatment with cannulated screws compared with treatment with Herbert screws. *J Bone Joint Surg Am* 1996;78:1829-1837.

86. Gelberman RH, Wolock BS, Siegel DB: Fractures and nonunions of the carpal scaphoid. *J Bone Joint Surg Am* 1989;71:1560-1565.

87. Mack GR, Bosse MJ, Gelberman RH, Yu E: The natural history of scaphoid non-union. *J Bone Joint Surg Am* 1984;66:504-509.

88. Lindstrom G, Nystrom A: Incidence of post-traumatic arthrosis after primary healing of scaphoid fractures: A clinical and radiological study. *J Hand Surg Br* 1990;15:11-13.

89. Ruby LK; Stinson J, Belsky MR: The natural history of scaphoid non-union: A review of fifty-five cases. *J Bone Joint Surg Am* 1985;67:428-432.

CHAPTER 2

THE ANATOMY OF THE SCAPHOID

RICHARD A. BERGER, MD, PHD

The scaphoid bone is the largest carpal bone in the proximal carpal row. Historically, it has been referred to as the *os naviculare*, or *navicular*, which is derived from the Latin diminutive form of *navis*, meaning ship, or *navicularis*, meaning of or related to shipping. These terms today have largely been abandoned as they relate to the wrist, rather reserving this name of the *tarsal navicular*. In keeping with a nautical theme, *scaphoid* is derived from the Greek word *skaphe*, meaning skiff or boat. This may even be related to the use of the term *carpus*, derived from the Greek root *karpos*, meaning a wharf. As will be seen, the shape of the scaphoid may in fact resemble, although quite loosely, the shape of a small boat hull. Regardless of semantics, the scaphoid is a fascinating structure; the mechanical integrity of the entire carpus depends on it. The geometry of the bone shares characteristics with contiguous elements in both the proximal and distal carpal rows and indeed appears to form a mechanical link between the carpal rows. It serves as the lateral column in the proximal carpal row arch. It also serves as a focus of ligamentous attachment and represents one of two areas in the proximal carpal row, along with the pisiform, that is dynamically influenced by extrinsic musculotendinous structures.

The carpal scaphoid is represented in some form in all mammals; however, in many it is found fused with the lunate to form the scapholunate bone or radiocarpal bone. In humans, the scaphoid seems particularly prone to injury, either as an isolated fracture or part of a ligamentous disruption pattern. Because of its unique anatomy and critical role in the wrist mechanics, such disruptions are often devastating to the function and long-term prognosis of the carpus if left uncompensated. Until the anatomy of the scaphoid and its role in the mechanical integrity of the wrist is fully understood, the chances of successfully treating patients with scaphoid pathology is measurably reduced. It is with this in mind that this chapter has been written.

OSSEOUS ANATOMY

The scaphoid has a complex three-dimensional geometry, which has been conveniently divided into three basic regions: proximal pole, waist, and distal pole (**Figure 1**). No specific landmarks have been agreed upon to objectively define the transitions between the regions. However, again by convention, the length of the scaphoid can simply be divided into thirds. Overall, the scaphoid has a palmar concave and medial (ulnar) concave curvature. Recent studies on the angulation of the body of the scaphoid have used landmarks established by the proximal and distal poles.[1] Using reference planes established by the palmar cortical surface of the proximal scaphoid and the dorsal cortical surface of the distal scaphoid, the intrascaphoid angle averaged 40° ± 3° in the coronal plane and 32° ± 5° in the sagittal plane. Varying the technique of measurement, using an estimate of the orientation of the proximal articular surface relative to the distal articular surface, the angulation between the axes averaged 24° ± 5° in the sagittal plane and 40° ± 4° in the coronal plane.

The proximal pole is defined as the area encompassed by articular cartilage, including the articular facet for

FIGURE 1

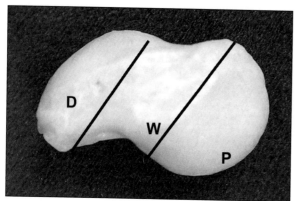

Right scaphoid from a dorsoradial perspective. The scaphoid is divided into three regions by its articular surfaces: proximal pole (P), waist (W, extra-articular), and distal pole (D). (Reproduced with permission from the Mayo Foundation.)

the lunate and the proximal articular surface (**Figure 2, A and B**). The articular surfaces for the trapezium and trapezoid (**Figure 2, C**), as well as the articular surface for the capitate, define the distal pole as far proximally as the extent of the tubercle on the palmar surface of the scaphoid (**Figure 2, D**). The entire expanse of scaphoid between these two regions is referred to as the waist. The articular surfaces are described in detail below.

The waist of the scaphoid has several consistent landmarks. First, there is a dorsal ridge extending nearly along the long axis of the scaphoid (**Figure 3**), which corresponds with the attachment of a reflection of the dorsal joint capsule. Just distal to the distal extent of the articular surface of the proximal pole, on the radial cortex of the waist, is a roughened area for attachment of the radial-most fibers of the radioscaphocapitate ligament. There are several foramina in this region where the dorsoradial nutrient vessels from either the radial artery proper of the dorsal radiocarpal arch perforate. Just distal to this region, without a clear demarcation, is the lateral cortex of the distal pole. It is here that the V-shaped scaphotrapezium ligament complex attaches and distal nutrient vessel foramina are found.[2] The palmar cortex of the waist is lined by the epiligamentous sheath of the radioscaphocapitate ligament proximally and distally serves as an attachment region of the central fibers of that same ligament.[3] The medial cortex of the waist is entirely covered in articular cartilage, serving as part

of the concave articular fossa for the head of the capitate.

ARTICULAR ANATOMY

Because of the unusual shape of the scaphoid, I have found it easier to describe details of surface anatomy in regions associated with specific articulations and ligaments. Such an approach is used in this discussion.

Articulation With the Radius

The surface area of the scaphoid that is available for articulation with the radius is second only to that region that articulates with the capitate. The region of the scaphoid from the most proximal surface through the midpoint of the waist forms this articulation. It is largely convex, matching the concave surface of the scaphoid fossa of the distal radius. There is a distinct ridge formed at the transition of cartilage to bone dedicated to ligament attachment, with the cartilage surface more prominent than its counterpoint. This surface transits to the palmar surface of the proximal row imperceptibly. The palmar surface rests on the long radiolunate ligament and is completely covered by articular cartilage.

Articulation With the Lunate

The surface area of the scaphoid that articulates with the lunate is flat, shaped like a crescent with the concave perimeter facing distally, and on the lateral aspect of the proximal pole. The transition between the lateral and proximal surfaces of the scaphoid is interrupted by the attachment of the scapholunate interosseous ligament at the dorsal, proximal, and palmar edges. This leaves the distal edge completely covered in articular cartilage. Because the proximal region of the scapholunate interosseous ligament is composed of fibrocartilage, the transition between articular surfaces is somewhat less pronounced.

Articulation With the Capitate

The large distal-medial surface of the scaphoid is dedicated to articulation with the capitate. Largely concave, it accommodates the convex surface of the head of the capitate, creating (with the lunate) a formidable socket

FIGURE 2

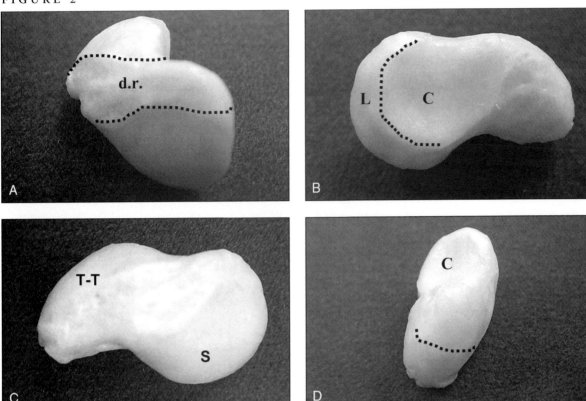

A, Right scaphoid from a proximodorsal perspective, demonstrating the proximal pole surface articulating with the scaphoid fossa of the distal radius, and the region of the dorsal ridge (dr). **B,** Medial surface of a right scaphoid demonstrating the articular fossa for the capitate (C) and the flat, crescentic articular surface for the lunate (L). **C,** Right scaphoid from a dorsoradial perspective demonstrating the articular regions for the scaphoid fossa of the radius (S) and the trapezium-trapezoid complex (T-T). **D,** Distal pole of a right scaphoid from a distal perspective. The capitate fossa (C) is visible over the dorsal edge of the distal pole. Note the different orientations of the articular surfaces for the trapezium and trapezoid, often separated by a subtle ridge (dotted line).(Reproduced with permission from the Mayo Foundation.)

for the capitate. At approximately the transition between the proximal pole and the waist of the scaphoid, there may be what appears to be a vertical crease in the articular surface. This corresponds to a relatively sharp transition in the articular surface of the head of the capitate between the proximal and lateral surfaces. A second vertical demarcation may be found in the central aspect of the waist of the scaphoid, corresponding to the transition from the head to the neck regions of the scaphoid.

Articulation With the Trapezoid and Trapezium

The distal surface of the scaphoid that articulates with the proximal surfaces of the trapezoid and trapezium is ellipsoid-to-rectangular in shape with the long axis oriented dorsopalmarly. Often, there is a slight difference in the planar orientation of the region articulating with the trapezoid relative to the region articulating with the trapezium, with the lateral being more perpendicular to the long axis of the scaphoid. If sufficient differences in orientation exist, a cartilage-covered edge may be appreciated at the transition between the surfaces. The transition between the distal and lateral surfaces is sharply demarcated, but covered in articular cartilage.

LIGAMENTOUS ATTACHMENTS

The scaphoid serves at an attachment surface for a number of important ligaments. First, along the dorsal, prox-

FIGURE 3

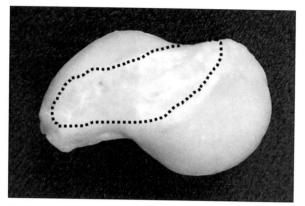

Right scaphoid from a dorsoradial perspective demonstrating the dorsoradial ridge (area within dotted line). (Reproduced with permission from the Mayo Foundation.)

FIGURE 4

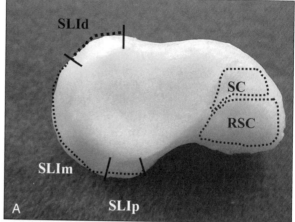

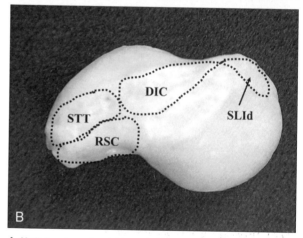

A, Medial surface of a right scaphoid demonstrating the attachment zones of the scaphocapitate ligament (SC), radioscaphocapitate ligament (RSC), and the dorsal (SLId), membranous (SLIm), and palmar (SLIp) regions of the scapholunate interosseous ligament. **B,** Right scaphoid from a dorsoradial perspective demonstrating the attachment zones of the scaphotrapezium-trapezoid ligament (STT), radioscaphocapitate ligament (RSC), dorsal intercarpal ligament (DIC), and the dorsal region of the scapholunate interosseous ligament (SLId). (Reproduced with permission from the Mayo Foundation.)

imal, and palmar edges of the medial edge of the proximal pole are the insertion zones for the three similarly named regions of the scapholunate interosseous ligament (**Figure 4**).[4] The radioscapholunate ligament, actually an extension of mesocapsule, inserts into the scapholunate interosseous ligament, rather than into the scaphoid itself. The long radiolunate ligament passes palmar to the proximal pole on its way to the lateral edge of the palmar surface of the lunate, anterior to the palmar region of the scapholunate interosseous ligament (**Figure 5**).[3] It does not insert directly into the scaphoid but often shares the epiligamentous sheath with the anterior surface of the proximal pole of the scaphoid as a periosteal reflection. The radioscaphocapitate ligament has substantial insertions into the scaphoid.[3] The most radial fibers attach to the lateral surface of the waist of the scaphoid, just distal to the edge of the articular cartilage of the proximal pole. The central aspect of the radioscaphocapitate ligament forms a V to surround and insert into the proximal surface of the distal pole. The remainder of the radioscaphocapitate ligament passes ulnarly anterior to the waist of the scaphoid to form part of the midcarpal joint palmar capsule.

Attaching to the lateral surface of the distal pole of the scaphoid is the scaphotrapezium ligament, forming a V ligament with its apex on the scaphoid.[2] This area also serves as an attachment of the proximal half of the dorsal intercarpal ligament.[5] The scaphocapitate ligament attaches to the palmar and lateral nonarticular surface of the distal pole of the scaphoid.

MUSCLE, TENDON, AND TENDON SHEATH ANATOMY

The tendon of flexor carpi ulnaris may have an influence on the scaphoid by virtue of the fibro-osseous tunnel that it passes through on the distal pole (**Figure 5**). This fibro-osseous tunnel continues to the trapezium. It is formed directly on the anterior surface of the

FIGURE 5

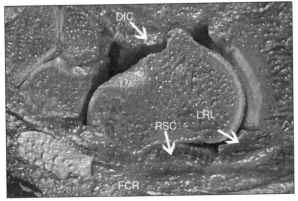

Cadaver specimen sagittally sectioned through the scaphoid. The dorsal intercarpal ligament (DIC) is seen in cross section just ulnar to its attachment to the dorsoradial ridge. The radioscaphocapitate ligament (RSC) inserts heavily into the palmar cortex of the waist of the scaphoid. Just proximal to the RSC ligament is the long radiolunate ligament (LRL), which has no attachment to the scaphoid. The tendon of flexor carpi radialis (FCR) passes palmar to the distal pole of the scaphoid through a fibro-osseous tunnel. (Reproduced with permission from the Mayo Foundation.)

FIGURE 6

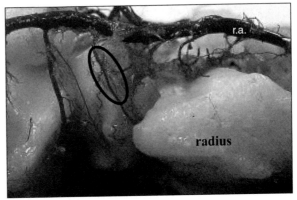

Cadaver prepared by injecting a polymer into the arterial tree and digesting all soft tissues. The radial artery (ra) branches into the dorsal intercarpal arch, which provides the nutrient vessels to the waist of the scaphoid (oval). Note the arterial concentration in the region of the scapholunate joint. (Reproduced with permission from the Mayo Foundation.)

distal pole and integrates with the scaphotrapezium and scaphocapitate ligaments. There is no formal ligamentous structure on the anterior surface of the scaphotrapezium joint. There are no analogous structures on the lateral or posterior surfaces of the scaphoid, although it is conceivable that the extensor carpi radialis brevis and longus provide some degree of reinforcement to the posterior wrist joint capsule immediately overlying the scaphoid.

VASCULAR ANATOMY

The blood supply to the scaphoid is divided into extraosseous and intraosseous categories to be completely understood. As with all living bones, nutrient arteries enter the cortex of the bone, forming the extraosseous supply. From here, internal vessels within the medullary chamber form the identifiable intraosseous supply, which ultimately arborizes into the haversian canal system, providing capillary-level vasculature.

The extraosseous blood supply is primarily derived from the radial artery and its branches, although indirectly, the high degree of anastomoses in the capsular

arches provides a redundancy of extraosseous blood supply potential from as far away as the ulnar artery and its branches (**Figure 6**). Gelberman and associates[6] and Taleisnik and Kelly[7] have identified three potential sources of extraosseous blood supply to the scaphoid. The distal pole is richly vascularized by nutrient vessels directly from the radial artery, entering into the lateral surface. Just proximal to this, at the level of the waist, are the dorsoradial vessels, typically originating from the radiocarpal or intercarpal arches in the dorsal wrist joint capsule. These vessels penetrate the scaphoid through the lateral surface of the waist and the dorsal ridge of the scaphoid, within the capsular reflection and progress proximally.[1,8,9] Few data suggest that a significant and consistent blood supply reaches the scaphoid through the scapholunate interosseous ligament.

PALPABLE ANATOMY

The ability to perform a physical examination with specificity and sensitivity is critical for the diagnosis of scaphoid fractures. Radiographs should be ordered to confirm the presence and define the type of fracture. However, this is strictly dependent upon the examiner's knowledge of underlying anatomy. The proximal pole, waist, and distal pole each can be specifically palpated on a routine physical examination of the wrist.

FIGURE 7

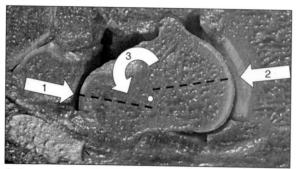

Cadaver specimen sagitally sectioned through the scaphoid demonstrating the offset proximal and distal articular surfaces. Loading of these surfaces produces a flexion moment of the scaphoid. 1= Force from radioscaphoid articulation; 2= Force transmitted through trapezium/trapezoid-scaphoid articulation; 3= Resultant moment on scaphoid. (Reproduced with permission from the Mayo Foundation.)

Proximal Pole

The proximal pole is palpable only from the dorsum of the wrist. It is easily found by first locating Lister's tubercle, the dorsal radial tubercle dividing the second and third extensor compartments. Palpating immediately distal to Lister's tubercle, the sulcus formed by the radiocarpal joint is palpated, and immediately distal to this is the prominence created by the scapholunate joint. Moving slightly lateral (radial) to this level places the examiner's finger on the proximal pole of the scaphoid.

Waist

The waist of the scaphoid can be palpated either dorsally or laterally. The dorsal surface of the waist can be found by palpating along and just distal to the dorsal rim of the distal radius toward the radial styloid process.

The lateral aspect of the waist can be palpated by entering the anatomic snuffbox. The anatomic snuffbox is defined as a triangular region between the radial styloid process, the tendon of extensor pollicis brevis, and the tendon of extensor pollicis longus. Deep within the anatomic snuffbox, the radial artery can be palpated, which defines the level of the scaphotrapezium joint. Moving proximally, in a neutrally positioned wrist, the distal pole of the scaphoid is palpated. By ulnarly deviating the wrist, the waist of the scaphoid is brought into the realm of the examiner's finger.

Distal Pole

The distal pole of the scaphoid can be palpated on its dorsal, lateral (radial), and palmar surfaces. The dorsal surface is found distal to the waist, essentially in the sulcus formed by the scaphotrapezoid joint. This interval is best appreciated between the tendons of extensor pollicis longus and extensor carpi radialis longus.

The lateral surface of the distal pole of the scaphoid is palpated as described for palpation of the waist of the scaphoid. The lateral aspect of the distal pole of the scaphoid is found just proximal to the radial artery as it crosses the anatomic snuffbox.

The palmar surface of the distal pole of the scaphoid is palpated through the tendon of flexor carpi radialis. The tendon enters a fibro-osseous tunnel based on the scaphoid and trapezium. The tendon is palpated as it crosses the wrist flexion crease. As the examiner's finger moves distally, the tendon suddenly becomes indistinct as a subcutaneous cord. It is at this point that the tendon has entered the fibro-osseous tunnel and hence marks the palmar surface of the distal pole of the scaphoid.

MECHANICS

In the truest sense of the word, the scaphoid provides a mechanical link between the proximal and distal rows. As elsewhere in this monograph, indirect proof of the linkage offered by the scaphoid is found in displaced fractures involving the proximal half of the scaphoid. In this scenario, the distal half behaves as a member of the distal carpal row, and the proximal fragment behaves as a member of the proximal carpal row. The shape of the scaphoid is such that the center of the distal articular surface is anterior to the center of the proximal articular surface. Thus, longitudinal loading of the scaphoid produces a flexion moment (**Figure 7**). The scalar value of this moment can be calculated as $M = Fd$, where M is the resultant moment, F is the magnitude of the force applied, and d is the perpendicular moment arm, defined as the distance between the point of force application and the axis of rotation. Thus, a flexion moment is generated and maximized by the distance (essentially the entire length of the scaphoid) between the scaphotrapezium-trapezoid ligament joint and the axis of flexion-extension in the proximal pole. This flexion moment is countered statically by the constraining ligaments at

---

TABLE 1

Rotational Displacement of the Scaphoid Relative to the Radius During Wrist Motion

	N-E^{60}	N-E^{30}	N-F^{30}	N-F^{60}
X axis rotation (+) pronation (-) supination	-2.5±3.4	-0.7±2.6	1.6±2.2	2.0±3.1
Y axis rotation (+) flexion (-) extension	-52.3±3.0	-26.0±3.2	20.6±2.8	39.7±4.3
Z axis rotation (+) ulnar deviation (-) radial deviation	4.5±3.7	0.8±2.1	2.1±2.2	7.8±4.5

Units are degrees with standard deviations.
N-E^{30} = neutral to 30° extension; N-E^{60} = neutral to 60° extension; N-F^{30} = neutral to 30° flexion; N=F^{60} = neutral to 60° flexion.[12]

---

the proximal and distal aspects of the scaphoid, and dynamically through the flexor carpi radialis tendon.

The kinematics of the scaphoid have been studied extensively.[10-12] As a generalization, displacement of the scaphoid during any finite range of wrist motion exceeds that of the triquetrum and lunate. During wrist flexion and extension motion, the scaphoid exhibits less motion than the capitate (Table 1). As the wrist progresses from flexion to extension, the scaphoid demonstrates supination; the opposite is seen during wrist flexion. During wrist radial deviation, the scaphoid exhibits primarily a flexion rotation, with a variable degree of ulnar translation. The scaphoid extends during ulnar deviation. The same pattern of pronation of the scaphoid is demonstrated during wrist radial deviation as it does during palmar flexion, and conversely it supinates during wrist ulnar deviation as it does during wrist dorsiflexion. Recently, a great deal of attention has been given to the kinematics of the wrist related to the "dart throw" axis. It has been determined in vivo that scaphoid and lunate motion is significantly less when following the dart throw path compared with the more cardinal paths of flexion-extension and radial-ulnar deviation.[13] It is entirely possible to envision a situation in which the scaphoid is locked into the scaphoid fossa and constrained by the radiocarpal and scapholunate ligament systems. Add to this a wrist position that is maximally extended and ulnarly deviated, out of the dart throw plane. Finally, add a direct, longitudinally oriented blow in which the additional forces applied are proportionately magnified through the moment concept, resulting in either a scaphoid fracture or a scapholunate dissociation.

CONCLUSION

The scaphoid is a critical link in the mechanism of the carpus. Its complex shape allows it to participate in the kinematics of both the proximal and distal rows. Because of its offset proximal and distal articular surfaces, it has a natural tendency to palmar flex with longitudinal loading. Because of this, extension of the scaphoid places progressively increasing tension on the palmar cortex of the curved waist of the scaphoid. Excessive extension, ulnar deviation, or both, of the wrist coupled with excessive loading mechanically predisposes the scaphoid to fracture. This is especially true if the strong ligaments attaching to the scaphoid hold their integrity. When a fracture occurs proximal to the waist of the scaphoid, it is predisposed to displacement because of the opposing forces on the proximal and distal fragments as well as the distribution of ligament attachments. This in turn predisposes the proximal fragment to ischemic conditions as a results of the distal location of nutrient vessels and a retrograde intraosseous blood supply.

REFERENCES

1. Smith DK, Linscheid RL, Amadio PC, Berquist TH, Cooney WP: Scaphoid anatomy: Evaluation with complex motion tomography. *Radiology* 1989;173:177-180.

2. Bettinger PC, Linscheid RL, Berger RA, Cooney WP, An K-N: An anatomic study of the stabilizing ligaments of the trapezium and trapziometacarpal joint. *J Hand Surg Am* 1999;24:786-798.

3. Berger RA, Landsmeer JMF: The palmar radiocarpal ligaments: A study of adult and fetal human wrist joints. *J Hand Surg Am* 1990;15:847-854.

4. Berger RA: The gross and histologic anatomy of the scapholunate interosseous ligament. *J Hand Surg Am* 1996;21:170-178.

5. Viegas SF, Yamaguchi S, Boyd NL, Patterson RM: The dorsal ligaments of the wrist: Anatomy, mechanical properties and function. *J Hand Surg* 1999;24:456-468.

6. Gelberman RH, Panagis JS, Taleisnik J, Baumgaertner M: The arterial anatomy of the human carpus: Part I. The extraosseous vascularity. *J Hand Surg Am* 1983;8:367-375.

7. Taleisnik J, Kelly PJ: The extraosseous and intraosseous blood supply of the scaphoid bone. *J Bone Joint Surg Am* 1966;48:1125-1137.

8. Gelberman RH, Menon J: The vascularity of the scaphoid bone. *J Hand Surg* 1980;5:508-513.

9. Panagis JS, Gelberman RH, Taleisnik J, Baumgaertner M: The arterial anatomy of the human carpus: Part II. The intraosseous vascularity. *J Hand Surg Am* 1983;8:375-382.

10. Berger RA, Crowninshield RD, Flatt AE: The three-dimensional rotational behaviors of the carpal bones. *Clin Orthop Rel Res* 1982;167:303-310.

11. Kobayashi M, Berger RA, Linscheid RL, An K-N: Intercarpal kinematics during wrist motion. *Hand Clin* 1997;13:143-149.

12. Kobayashi M, Berger RA, Nagy L, et al: Normal kinematics of carpal bones: A three-dimensional analysis of carpal bone motion relative to the radius. *J Biomech* 1997;30:787-793.

13. Crisco JJ, Coburn JC, Moore DC, Akelman E, Weiss AP, Wolfe SW: In vivo radiocarpal kinematics and the dart thrower's motion. *J Bone Joint Surg Am* 2005;87:2729-2740.

CHAPTER 3

CHALLENGES IN IMAGING SCAPHOID FRACTURES

KIMBERLY K. AMRAMI, MD

The scaphoid is the most commonly fractured of the carpal bones.[1] Scaphoid fractures most commonly occur in active young adults but rarely in children or the elderly.[2] They are significant because of their potential complications, including nonunion or delayed union, osteonecrosis (ON), and osteoarthritis.[1,2] All of these complications are more likely with delays in diagnosis and treatment.

RADIOGRAPHY

When patients present to the emergency department with snuffbox tenderness after a fall on an outstretched hand, a scaphoid fracture is the most important consideration; however, other injuries, such as Colles' and radial styloid fractures or even soft-tissue injuries of the first extensor compartment, may have similar clinical presentations.[1,3] The first step in imaging always should be well-positioned posteroanterior (PA) and lateral radiographs.[4] It is especially important that the PA view be obtained with the wrist in a neutral position without significant radial deviation and scaphoid flexion, which may simulate pathology. In many situations, a wrist trauma series also includes a PA view of the wrist in ulnar deviation to fully extend the scaphoid, potentially making fractures at the scaphoid waist easier to visualize. A recent study retrospectively reviewed radiographs obtained in 113 patients with scaphoid fractures that had been identified on radiography.[5] There was no cross-sectional correlation. The authors assessed the views obtained and the clarity of depiction of the fracture on each type of image. They found that all scaphoid fractures that could be seen on elongated and supinated oblique views also could be seen on other views and concluded that the minimum radiographic examination for a suspected scaphoid fracture should include PA, lateral, pronated oblique, and ulnar-deviated PA views. The authors specifically noted that fractures through the proximal third of the scaphoid might be seen only on the pronated oblique view.

MAGNETIC RESONANCE IMAGING

In addition to actually visualizing a fracture on radiograph, it has long been purported that secondary signs of fracture such as an obscured or displaced radiolucent fat stripe adjacent to the scaphoid on the PA radiograph adjacent to the waist of the scaphoid are sensitive signs of scaphoid fracture. A retrospective study of 78 confirmed scaphoid fractures identified an abnormal scaphoid fat stripe in 73 of 78 radiographs.[6] However, more recent studies have shown that this is an inconsistent finding, with only about 50% sensitivity and specificity for a scaphoid fracture that could be seen on MRI.[7] In addition to the poor accuracy for the presence of a fracture, a positive fat stripe sign was present in 30% of patients without a scaphoid fracture, making the presence or absence of the fat stripe a poor predictor for an underlying radiographically occult fracture.[7,8]

Unfortunately, radiography may fail to demonstrate a nondisplaced fracture even when well positioned and interpreted by an expert observer. Cooney[9] estimated that up to 40% of scaphoid fractures remain undiagnosed at the time of injury. Even when appropriate care is sought and radiographs are obtained, a significant proportion of scaphoid fractures are missed. Initial radiographs demonstrate a fracture in 70% to 90% of patients.[10,11] A meta-analysis of studies assessing at the accuracy of MRI for scaphoid fractures reported that up to 16% of fractures were radiographically occult.[12] In addition, interobserver reliability for detection of scaphoid fractures on radiography is poor, with a ê value of only 0.4 on a study that reviewed radiographs at the time of injury and then at 2 and 6 weeks by four readers of varying experience.[13] Considering that as many as 36% of patients in whom scaphoid fractures are suspected actually have them, this becomes a significant number in which the diagnosis is missed or delayed.[1] Conversely, patients without scaphoid fracture may unnecessarily undergo immobilization when clinical symptoms are present even without objective diagnostic proof.[14] In the words of Barton,[15] "we overtreat a lot of patients to avoid undertreating a few."

Computed Tomography

At the time of initial evaluation, scaphoid fractures can be divided into two categories: those that are visible on radiographs and those that are radiographically occult. Radiographically visible fractures are typically evaluated with CT as part of the decision-making process for treatment.[16] Desai and associates[17] looked at radiographic characteristics of scaphoid fractures using the Herbert, Compson, and Russe classification systems and found poor inter- and intraobserver reliability and impressively diverse assessments of displacement with no correlation with these features and later fracture union. With its multiplanar capabilities and high spatial resolution, CT easily identifies comminution, displacement, and alignment and can be performed with the patient in a cast or with fixation hardware in place.[18,19] Three-dimensional reconstructions are widely available, allowing for visualization of the entire wrist as well as individual bones and articular surfaces, making it ideal for surgical planning. In addition, MRI can be used for this purpose,[20] but CT generally has been used in the situations in which a fracture is visualized radiographically and further assessment is desired.

Other Imaging Modalities

In cases where scaphoid fracture is suspected and radiographs are negative or equivocal, several approaches have been suggested.[4] One option is to immobilize patients with a presumptive diagnosis of scaphoid fracture and to obtain additional images in some follow-up time period, typically between 2 and 6 weeks.[8,21,22] The theory behind this practice is that bone resorption around the fracture makes it more visible. A recent study reviewed 50 sets of radiographs at the time of injury and then at 10 to 50 days later.[22] All initial radiographs had been judged normal at the time of injury. The radiographs were reviewed in a blinded fashion by four reviewers, including specialists from emergency medicine, hand surgery, and radiology. Each patient also had an MRI obtained on a low-field dedicated extremity magnet as the gold standard for diagnosis. Of the 50 patients, 35 had scaphoid fractures, and 15 had no fracture. For the follow-up radiograph, individual observers had a sensitivity of 11% to 43%, with specificities for all in the 90th percentile but negative predictive values only as high as 40%. Furthermore, the interobserver reliability was very poor at only 33%. Thus, relying on follow-up radiographs to diagnose scaphoid fractures that are occult on initial studies leaves us with the same dilemma present on evaluation of the initial studies—there is a significant risk of missing a fracture and an increased risk of late complications.

Other imaging studies are available to evaluate patients in whom scaphoid fracture is suspected but radiographs are equivocal or normal, including scintigraphy (bone scan), MRI, CT, and more recently ultrasound. Polytomography, a mainstay in the past for this purpose, is no longer available and has been effectively replaced by CT.

Scintigraphy

Scintigraphy has been considered to have near-perfect sensitivity for occult fractures, and advocates claim that this should be the second study in this clinical setting.[9,23] Unfortunately, specificity is low, with up to 25% false-positive results using follow-up radiographs as a guide.[24] Recent studies have suggested this is a fast and reliable diagnostic tool, but imaging in the delayed phase requires at least a 3-hour wait after injection, and clin-

FIGURE 1

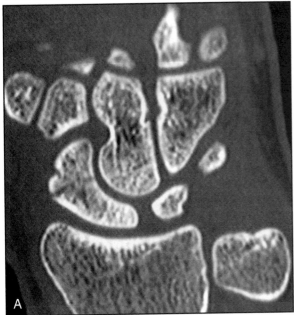 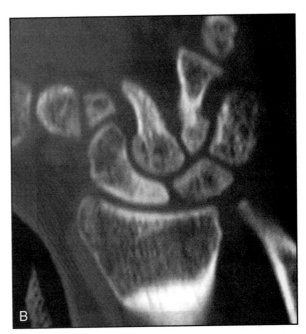

A, Coronal reformatted CT scan of the wrist on an eight-row MDCT system. Note the crisp definition of the scaphoid waist fracture. **B,** Follow-up examination performed on a four-row MDCT system. Note the slight blurring of trabecular detail compared with **(A).**

ical guidelines suggest that patients wait at least 72 hours after the initial injury before undergoing scintigraphy to avoid early false-negative results.[23] Groves and associates[25] report increased detection of scaphoid fractures on scintigraphy compared with multidetector CT (MDCT), but follow-up radiographs and MRI scans in 7 of 23 patients failed to show fractures. These discordant cases did have quantitatively lower uptake of the radiotracer than the concordant fractures, and the authors concluded that these may represent bone contusions rather than complete fractures. In a study comparing scintigraphy and MRI in 40 patients (six proven scaphoid fractures), there were two false-positive and one false-negative bone scans, with no misses or overcalls on MRI.[4] These results confirm the impression of other investigators, namely, scintigraphy is sensitive but not specific in the detection of scaphoid fractures.

Computed Tomography

Computed tomography is another modality that has been proposed for the investigation of clinically suspected but radiographically occult scaphoid fractures.

CT is widely available and usually can be obtained at all hours of the day and night. The advent of MDCT has led to increasing spatial resolution and enhanced multiplanar capabilities (**Figure 1**). Unfortunately, CT has sensitivity lower than either scintigraphy or MRI for the diagnosis of scaphoid fractures. A study of 51 patients with suspected wrist fractures compared state-of-the-art CT (16-row MDCT) with high-resolution scintigraphy.[26] There was discordance in 13.7% of patients; CT identified 27% of fractures and bone scan, 45%. In the seven discordant cases in which the bone scan was positive and CT negative, repeat studies at 6 weeks showed fractures in only three patients, demonstrating both the high sensitivity and low specificity of bone scan and the relatively low sensitivity and specificity of CT in this setting. In addition to a case report from the same group,[27] a study comparing CT and MRI showed two false-negative examinations out of a total of 18 fractures seen on MRI.[28] A single small study of 29 patients with seven identified scaphoid fractures reported 100% sensitivity and specificity for CT for scaphoid fractures, but there was no comparison with MRI or any follow-up of these patients with scintigraphy considered the gold standard,

FIGURE 2

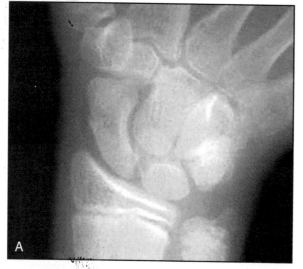

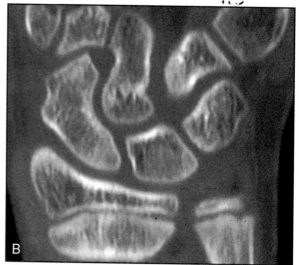

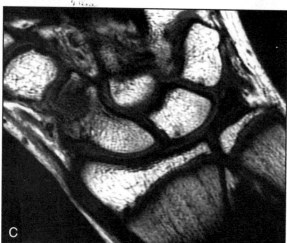

A, Photographic enlargement of a PA radiograph in ulnar deviation of a 14-year-old boy with anatomic snuffbox tenderness after he injured his forearm on his motorbike handlebars. No fracture is seen, and the normal fat stripe adjacent to the waist of the scaphoid is present. **B,** CT scan with coronal reformatting obtained 1 day later is negative for fracture. **C,** Coronal T1-weighted MRI scan obtained immediately after CT shows a comminuted fracture at the waist of the scaphoid, which was occult on both radiography and CT.

even though the investigators report both false-positive and false-negative scintigraphy results.[29] A study performed specifically to compare CT and MRI included 52 consecutive patients with suspected scaphoid fracture showed fractures in 18 detected by a limited protocol on a low-field MRI, but only 16 were seen on multiplanar CT.[28] Looking at all of these results, we can conclude that if CT is used to further evaluate a patient with a suspected scaphoid fractures and negative radiographs, the question remains unresolved in up to 13% of patients (**Figure 2**).

Ultrasound

Several investigators have suggested the use of ultrasound for the diagnosis of scaphoid fractures.[30-34] Early reports using very-low-frequency transducers indicated that ultrasound was not helpful[35] for diagnosing scaphoid fractures, but more recent reports using high-frequency transducers (>10 MHz) and high-resolution imaging report sensitivity for fractures ranging from 78% to 100%, depending on whether the diagnostic criteria such as definitive identification of cortical disrup-

FIGURE 3

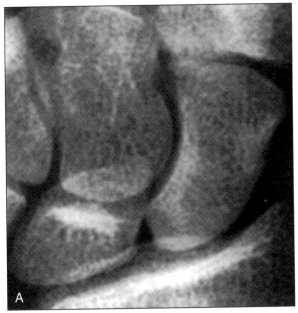 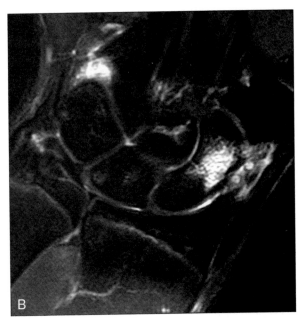

A, Enlarged PA radiograph of the wrist obtained in a 20-year-old man 3 days after he fell on his outstretched hand. There is questionable cortical irregularity at the scaphoid tubercle, but the normal fat stripe is present, and the examination was read as normal. **B,** T2-weighted coronal MRI scan with fat suppression obtained 1 day later shows a complete and nondisplaced scaphoid waist fracture with disruption of both cortices.

tion were strictly applied.[33,34] In one study, ultrasound was less sensitive and specific than radiography,[32] but another study showed only one false-positive result out of five patients and no false negatives.[33] A study in which CT was used as the gold standard had 100% sensitivity and 79% specificity for high-resolution sonography (7 to 15 MHz) compared with CT, but included only five fractures.[34] This discordance between studies and sites may be related to an inherent weakness of musculoskeletal ultrasound: it is profoundly operator and experience dependent. Ultrasound may have a role in the diagnosis of radiographically occult scaphoid fractures in the future, but the technique is not sufficiently developed at this time to be a good screening tool.

ADVANTAGES OF MRI

The preferred second-line test is MRI for the evaluation of scaphoid fractures in patients with negative radiographs (**Figure 3**). Sensitivity has been reported in the 95% to 100% range, and specificity is consistently

reported at 100%.[36] A negative MRI scan with no bone marrow edema is truly negative, and no further treatment is required. When individual imaging sequences are assessed, the most valuable are spin-echo T1- and fluid-sensitive T2-weighted sequences; these have the highest sensitivity and specificity and in combination have the highest accuracy. The lowest sensitivity is seen with T2 gradient echo images, which had a sensitivity for fracture of only 14% compared with 100% for short ô inversion recovery.[36] When strict diagnostic criteria are applied (identification of a low signal band on T1 images), accuracy improves even further. Interobserver reliability has been reported as nearly perfect ($\hat{e} = 0.953$), suggesting that this test is less dependent on the experience of the interpreting physician compared with the low inter- and intraobserver reliability for the diagnosis of scaphoid fractures on radiographs.[12,36]

Another advantage of MRI in the diagnosis of scaphoid fractures is that low-field and dedicated extremity scanners may be used for this purpose without any decrease in accuracy, making this test widely

FIGURE 4

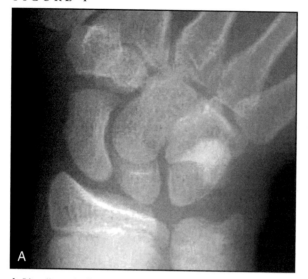 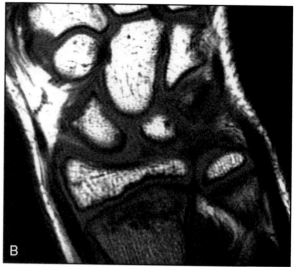

A, PA radiograph of the wrist of an 11-year-old boy after he injured the wrist on the playground. No fractures are seen. Snuffbox tenderness was present, and scaphoid fracture was the clinical diagnosis. **B**, T1-weighted coronal MRI scan of the wrist obtained the same day shows a nondisplaced comminuted fracture of the distal radius with extension along the physeal plate. The fracture was treated with closed reduction and healed uneventfully.

available in areas outside of large tertiary referral centers. Breitenseher and associates[37] compared a 0.2T in-office dedicated extremity scanner to a 1.0T whole body system with dedicated surface coils and found no difference in fracture diagnosis. Higher field imaging (>1.5T) improves the signal-to-noise ratio and may have a role where very strict diagnostic criteria requiring distinct cortical disruption are applied and high spatial resolution is a requirement. If both T1- and T2-weighted images with fat suppression are obtained in at least two planes, there should be no decrease in sensitivity using lower field systems. Contrast generally is not necessary, although its use has been reported to improve detection of fractures and to evaluate the vascularity of fracture fragments,[38] and there are no limitations such as age or reproductive status as long as criteria for MRI safety are met.

In addition, MRI is accurate in identifying other pathology that may present either in association with scaphoid fractures or mimicking its clinical presentation (**Figure 4**). In a large series reported by Brydie and Raby,[1] MRI was obtained in 195 patients with clinical findings suspicious for scaphoid fracture and negative radiographs. Ninety-nine (51%) patients had no frac-

ture, and 37 (19%) had scaphoid fractures. In addition to those findings, however, MRI identified 8 (4%) other carpal fractures and 28 (14.4%) fractures of the distal radius. In this prospective study, patient management was affected by the MRI results in 92%, and occult fractures were diagnosed in almost 40%. MRI also has been used to assess fracture displacement and alignment for treatment planning.[20] This study showed reasonable inter- and intraobserver reliability for fracture displacement and sagittal translation with accuracy of 1 to 2 mm, providing improved assessment of these parameters compared with plain radiographs. Of 49 fractures seen on follow-up, 3 failed to unite; all were displaced by more than 1 mm in the sagittal plane, suggesting that MRI may be used to assess likelihood of union, which could contribute to surgical decision making at the time of injury. Further studies are required before MRI can replace CT for surgical planning for these fractures.

In less experienced hands, MRI has limitations, and one of the most difficult is its extreme sensitivity to bone marrow edema.[16] One of the biggest difficulties in interpreting these examinations is trying to distinguish bone contusions or incomplete or microtrabecular fractures from complete but nondisplaced fractures (**Figure 5**).

The definitive proof may come only after a period of immobilization and the appearance of a discrete fracture line on follow-up radiographs.[27] This is certainly a pitfall of diagnosis, but with experience and dogmatic adherence to criteria requiring the identification of an actual fracture line, this generally may be avoided. In these instances, overtreating a small number of patients may be unavoidable, but it is hoped that the 80% to 85% overtreatment statistic, as reported by Gaebler and associates,[14] can be avoided when no advanced imaging modality is used for diagnosis and all patients with suspected fractures are treated with immobilization.

Cost is another significant consideration in imaging for suspected scaphoid fractures. Alternatives to MRI as a second-line test include office fluoroscopy, serial radiographs, scintigraphy, and CT. The actual cost of MRI in the United States is comparable to a bone scan or CT scan but considerably more than office fluoroscopy or follow-up radiographs. It is important to take into account more than the cost of the study itself when considering the actual economic impact of different algorithms for identifying patients with scaphoid fractures. Several studies performed in the United Kingdom and New Zealand and Australia report that the cost of overall care was reduced by using MRI for early diagnosis.[14,38-42] A more recent study from Australia showed an increase in health care-related charges when MRI was used for diagnosis, but this study did not account for productivity losses when unnecessary immobilization was used.[21] All of these countries have some form of national health care, which makes comparisons with North America in general and the United States in particular difficult, but a study including four patients done at a major academic institution in the United States showed the medical charges to be roughly equivalent for traditional treatment with follow-up and an abbreviated screening MRI with a limited charge.[43] A distinct advantage of MRI is that is has near-perfect specificity.[36] Because of this, MRI is the ideal test for excluding fractures that require treatment. The most substantial cost savings are seen in the ability to maintain employment and productivity when no fracture is present compared with costs for patients who undergo unnecessary treatments such as casting and splinting, which limit activity, and in accurately diagnosing other injuries, which may be treated differently.[15,41,44] The use of MRI in the acute setting has been advocated in a recent best-evi-

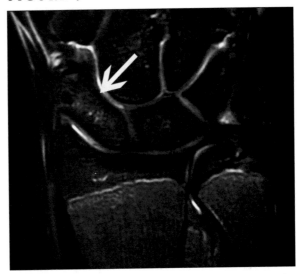

High-resolution 3T coronal T2-weighted MRI scan of the wrist with fat suppression shows indistinct increased T2 signal in the distal half of the scaphoid (arrow) consistent with a very mild contusion. There was no fracture; therefore, no treatment was required.

dence topic report that reviewed bone scintigraphy versus MRI; the report suggested that MRI is slightly superior for scaphoid fractures and had the advantage of identifying other bone and soft-tissue pathology accurately.[3] The authors also reported that the diagnosis was obtained more quickly, allowing for prompt and appropriate treatment.

Assessment of healing of scaphoid fractures after immobilization or internal fixation is best performed with high-resolution CT with multiplanar reformatting. This shows to best advantage bridging callus across the fracture or conversely the development of cortication of the nonunited fragments indicating a nonunion. For this purpose, MRI may be used with relatively little artifact related to hardware fixation (**Figure 6**),[6,45,46] but CT generally is preferred for both surgical planning and postoperative follow-up.[16,18,19] Doppler ultrasound[31] and MRI with dynamic contrast enhancement[47] have been used to assess fracture healing by looking at increased blood flow to the healing fracture, but these techniques have not been widely adopted.

In the first months of healing, radiography or CT may show increased density in the proximal portion of the scaphoid, but this may represent reactive change and not

FIGURE 6

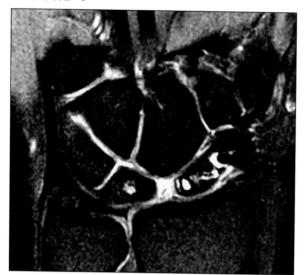

Coronal T2-weighted MRI scan of the wrist with fat suppression showing minimal artifact related to screw fixation of a scaphoid waist fracture and failed repair of an associated scapholunate ligament tear with suture anchors in the scaphoid and lunate. Note the healed scaphoid fracture and scapholunate dissociation.

FIGURE 7

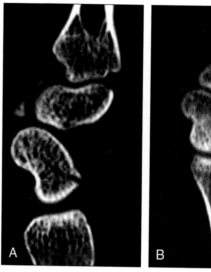

Sagittal reformatted CT images obtained 1 week (**A**) and 4 weeks (**B**) after scaphoid fracture. Note increased density in the proximal pole on (**B**) as well as the interval healing of the fracture. This was judged to be likely reactive and resolved without progression to ON.

necessarily be the harbinger of ON (**Figure 7**). Russe[48] reported increased density in up to 30% of healing scaphoid fractures with radiography and suggested that this was a transient phenomenon as a result of damage to nutrient vessels. Neither he nor later authors believed that increased density in the proximal pole fragment predicted healing or that there was an absolute relationship between increased density and low blood flow.[48,49] When ON is suspected, MRI is the preferred modality for confirmation with several grading systems available.[50-52] All are based on evaluation of the assessment of trabecular bone and signal changes in fatty marrow. Early on, there may be edema, which by itself is an insensitive sign; the most sensitive sign for ON on an unenhanced MRI is the loss of fatty marrow in the affected portion of bone.[50] This finding is commonly seen before changes can be perceived on CT or radiography and is more sensitive and specific than increased density in the proximal pole fragment. Other authors have distinguished between acute and chronic fractures, reporting that gadolinium-enhanced MRI was a valuable tool for prognostication, but these studies used delayed imaging and not dynamic enhancement.[53] Currently, there is no definitive answer as to the role of gadolinium-enhanced

MRI for predicting the risk of ON or treatment outcomes; published reports conflict.[38,47,54] In my practice, I occasionally use dynamic enhancement to assess proximal pole vascularity before surgical treatment with vascularized bone grafts. If flow is detected on the first enhancement phase (arterial), then a presumption can be made regarding an intact vascular supply; but there are no good scientific data to support this assumption. In a small series of 15 patients, MRI was used to assess the incorporation of vascularized bone grafts.[55] This study showed that MRI can assess graft incorporation, viability, and healing earlier than radiographs, potentially allowing earlier mobilization after surgery. Larger studies are needed to confirm this finding and to establish the role of MRI after vascularized bone graft for scaphoid nonunions.

Conclusion

Early diagnosis leading to effective and prompt treatment remains the goal for imaging injuries of the scaphoid. Radiography, scintigraphy, CT, and even ultrasound have all been proposed for early diagnosis of scaphoid fractures, but MRI remains the diagnostic study of choice for all fractures of the distal forearm and wrist that are not radiographically obvious. In addition to its high sensitivity and specificity for scaphoid fractures, MRI has the ability to identify a variety of other pathologies including fractures of the radius and other carpal bones, ligament injuries, and other problems that may present with similar symptoms. Despite its high cost, the use of MRI after an acute injury is the recommended second-line test after radiography for suspected scaphoid fractures. It ultimately is cost effective when the relationship between early diagnosis and treatment and the impact on lost productivity and decreased late complications is considered. For fractures visible on radiography, CT remains the imaging study of choice for surgical planning and assessment of healing after closed and open reduction. The use of advanced imaging studies for predicting outcomes of treatment for scaphoid fractures remains controversial, and further study is required before consensus on a best practice standard can be reached.

REFERENCES

1. Brydie A, Raby N: Early MRI in the management of clinical scaphoid fracture [see comment]. *Br J Radiol* 2003;76:296-300.

2. Phillips TG, Reibach AM, Slomiany WP: Diagnosis and management of scaphoid fractures. *Am Fam Phys* 2004;70:879-884.

3. Foex B, Speake P, Body R: Best evidence topic report: Magnetic resonance imaging or bone scintigraphy in the diagnosis of plain x-ray occult scaphoid fractures. *Emerg Med J* 2005;22:434-435.

4. Fowler C, Sullivan B, Williams LA, McCarthy G, Savage R, Palmer A: A comparison of bone scintigraphy and MRI in the early diagnosis of the occult scaphoid waist fracture. *Skeletal Radiol* 1998;27:683-687.

5. Cheung GC, Lever CJ, Morris AD: X-ray diagnosis of acute scaphoid fractures. *J Hand Surg Br* 2006;31:104-109.

6. Cetti R, Christensen SE: The diagnostic value of displacement of the fat stripe in fracture of the scaphoid bone. *Hand* 1982;14:75-79.

7. Annamalai G, Raby N: Scaphoid and pronator fat stripes are unreliable soft tissue signs in the detection of radiographically occult fractures [see comment]. *Clin Radiol* 2003;58:798-800.

8. Dias JJ, Finlay DB, Brenkel IJ, Gregg PJ: Radiographic assessment of soft tissue signs in clinically suspected scaphoid fractures: The incidence of false negative and false positive results. *J Orthop Trauma* 1987;1:205-208.

9. Cooney WP III: Scaphoid fractures: Current treatments and techniques. *Instr Course Lect* 2003;52:197-208.

10. Brondum V, Larsen CF, Skov O: Fracture of the carpal scaphoid: Frequency and distribution in a well-defined population. *Eur J Radiol* 1992;15:118-122.

11. Leslie IJ, Dickson RA: The fractured carpal scaphoid: Natural history and factors influencing outcome. *J Bone Joint Surg Br* 981;63:225-230.

12. Hunter JC, Escobedo EM, Wilson AJ, Hanel DP, Zink-Brody GC, Mann FA: MR imaging of clinically suspected scaphoid fractures. *AJR Am J Roentgenol* 1997;168:1287-1293.

13. Tiel-van Buul MM, van Beek EJ, Broekhuizen AH, Nooitgedacht EA, Davids PH, Bakker AJ: Diagnosing scaphoid fractures: Radiographs cannot be used as a gold standard! *Injury* 1992;23(2):77-79.

14. Gaebler C, Kukla C, Breitenseher M, Trattnig S, Mittlboeck M, Vecsei V: Magnetic resonance imaging of occult scaphoid fractures. *J Trauma* 1996;41:73-76.

15. Barton NJ: Twenty questions about scaphoid fractures. *J Hand Surg Br* 1992;17:289-310.

16. Krimmer H: Management of acute fractures and nonunions of the proximal pole of the scaphoid. *J Hand Surg Br* 2002;27:245-248.

17. Desai VV, Davis TR, Barton NJ: The prognostic value and reproducibility of the radiological features of the fractured scaphoid. *J Hand Surg Br* 1999;24:586-590.

18. Fayad LM, Bluemke DA, Fishman EK: Musculoskeletal imaging with computed tomography and magnetic resonance imaging: When is computed tomography the study of choice? *Curr Probl Diagn Radiol* 2005;34:220-237.

19. Bush CH, Gillespy T III, Dell PC: High-resolution CT of the wrist: Initial experience with scaphoid disorders and surgical fusions. *AJR Am J Roentgenol* 1987;149:757-760.

20. Bhat M, McCarthy M, Davis TR, Oni JA, Dawson S: MRI and plain radiography in the assessment of displaced fractures of the waist of the carpal scaphoid. *J Bone Joint Surg Br* 2004;86:705-713.

21. Brooks S, Wluka AE, Stuckey S, Cicuttini F: The management of scaphoid fractures. *J Sci Med Sport* 2005;8:181-189.

22. Low G, Raby N: Can follow-up radiography for acute scaphoid fracture still be considered a valid investigation? *Clin Radiol* 2005;60:1106-1110.

23. Beeres FJ, Hogervorst M, Hollander P, Rhemrev S: Outcome of routine bone scintigraphy in suspected scaphoid fractures. *Injury* 2005;36:1233-1236.

24. Tiel-van Buul MM, van Beek EJ, Broekhuizen AH, Bakker AJ, Bos KE, van Royen EA: Radiography and scintigraphy of suspected scaphoid fracture: A long-term study in 160 patients [see comment]. *J Bone Joint Surg Br* 1993;75:61-65.

25. Groves AM, Cheow HK, Balan KK, Bearcroft PW, Dixon AK: 16 detector multislice CT versus skeletal scintigraphy in the diagnosis of wrist fractures: Value of quantification of 99Tcm-MDP uptake. *Br J Radiol* 2005;78:791-795.

26. Groves AM, Cheow H, Balan K, Courtney H, Bearcroft P, Dixon A: 16-MDCT in the detection of occult wrist fractures: A comparison with skeletal scintigraphy. *AJR Am J Roentgenol* 2005;184:1470-1474.

27. Groves AM, Cheow HK, Balan KK, Courtney HM, Bearcroft PW, Dixon AK: Case report: False negative 16 detector multislice CT for scaphoid fracture. *Br J Radiol* 2005;78:57-59.

28. Kusano N, Churei Y, Shiraishi E, Kusano T: Diagnosis of occult carpal scaphoid fracture: A comparison of magnetic resonance imaging and computed tomography techniques. *Tech Hand Up Extrem Surg* 2002;6:119-123.

29. Breederveld RS, Tuinebreijer WE: Investigation of computed tomographic scan concurrent criterion validity in doubtful scaphoid fracture of the wrist. *J Trauma* 2004;57:851-854.

30. Herneth AM, Siegmeth A, Bader TR, et al: Scaphoid fractures: Evaluation with high-spatial-resolution US initial results. *Radiology* 2001;220:231-235.

31. Hodgkinson DW, Nicholson DA, Stewart G, Sheridan M, Hughes P: Scaphoid fracture: A new method of assessment. *Clin Radiol* 1993;48:398-401.

32. Senall JA, Failla JM, Bouffard JA, van Holsbeeck M: Ultrasound for the early diagnosis of clinically suspected scaphoid fracture. *J Hand Surg Am* 2004;29:400-405.

33. Hauger O, Bonnefoy O, Moinard M, Bersani D, Diard F: Occult fractures of the waist of the scaphoid: Early diagnosis by high-spatial-resolution sonography. *AJR Am J Roentgenol* 2002;178:1239-1245.

34. Fusetti C, Poletti PA, Pradel PH, et al: Diagnosis of occult scaphoid fracture with high-spatial-resolution sonography: A prospective blind study. *J Trauma* 2005;59:677-681.

35. Christiansen TG, Rude C, Lauridsen KK, Christensen OM: Diagnostic value of ultrasound in scaphoid fractures. *Injury* 1991;22:397-399.

36. Breitenseher MJ, Metz VM, Gilula LA, et al: Radiographically occult scaphoid fractures: Value of MR imaging in detection. *Radiology* 1997;203:245-250.

37. Breitenseher MJ, Trattnig S, Gabler C, et al: MRI in radiologically occult scaphoid fractures: Initial experiences with 1.0 Tesla (whole body-middle field equipment) versus 0.2 Tesla (dedicated low-field equipment) [in German]. *Radiologe* 1997;37:812-818.

38. Munk PL, Lee MJ, Janzen DL, et al: Gadolinium-enhanced dynamic MRI of the fractured carpal scaphoid: Preliminary results. *Australas Radiol* 1998;42:10-15.

39. Gooding A, Coates M, Rothwell A: Accident compensation C. Cost analysis of traditional follow-up protocol versus MRI for radiographically occult scaphoid fractures: A pilot study for the Accident Compensation Corporation. *N Z Med J* 2004;117:U1049.

40. Pillai A, Jain M: Management of clinical fractures of the scaphoid: Results of an audit and literature review. *Eur J Emerg Med* 2005;12:47-51.

41. Brooks S, Cicuttini FM, Lim S, Taylor D, Stuckey SL, Wluka AE: Cost effectiveness of adding magnetic resonance imaging to the usual management of suspected scaphoid fractures. *Br J Sports Med* 2005;39:75-79.

42. Moller JM, Larsen L, Bovin J, et al: MRI diagnosis of fracture of the scaphoid bone: Impact of a new practice where the images are read by radiographers. *Acad Radiol* 2004;11:724-728.

43. Dorsay TA, Major NM, Helms CA: Cost-effectiveness of immediate MR imaging versus traditional follow-up for revealing radiographically occult scaphoid fractures.[see comment]. *AJR Am J Roentgenol* 2001;177:1257-1263.

44. Saxena P, McDonald R, Gull S, Hyder N: Diagnostic scanning for suspected scaphoid fractures: An economic evaluation based on cost-minimization models. *Injury* 2003;34:503-511.

45. McNally EG, Goodman R, Burge P: The role of MRI in the assessment of scaphoid fracture healing: A pilot study. *Eur Radiol* 2000;10:1926-1928.

46. Morgan WJ, Breen TF, Coumas JM, Schulz LA: Role of magnetic resonance imaging in assessing factors affecting healing in scaphoid nonunions. *Clin Orthop Rel Res* 1997;336:240-246.

47. Dawson JS, Martel AL, Davis TR: Scaphoid blood flow and acute fracture healing: A dynamic MRI study with enhancement with gadolinium. *J Bone Joint Surg Br* 2001;83:809-814.

48. Russe O: Fracture of the carpal navicular. Diagnosis, non-operative treatment and operative treatment. *J Bone Joint Surg Am* 1960;42:759-768.

49. Downing ND, Oni JA, Davis TR, Vu TQ, Dawson JS, Martel AL: The relationship between proximal pole blood flow and the subjective assessment of increased

density of the proximal pole in acute scaphoid fractures. *J Hand Surgery Am* 2002;27:402-408.

50. Golimbu CN, Firooznia H, Rafii M: Avascular necrosis of carpal bones. *Magn Reson Imaging Clin North Am* 1995;3:281-303.

51. Schmitt R, Heinze A, Fellner F, Obletter N, Struhn R, Bautz W: Imaging and staging of avascular osteonecroses at the wrist and hand. *Eur J Radiol* 1997;25:92-103.

52. Chang MA, Bishop AT, Moran SL, Shin AY: The outcomes and complications of 1,2-intercompartmental supraretinacular artery pedicled vascularized bone grafting of scaphoid nonunions. *J Hand Surg Am* 2006;31:387-396.

53. Cerezal L, Abascal F, Canga A, Garcia-Valtuille R, Bustamante M, del Pinal F: Usefulness of gadolinium-enhanced MR imaging in the evaluation of the vascularity of scaphoid nonunions. *AJR Am J Roentgenol* 2000;174:141-149.

54. Singh AK, Davis TR, Dawson JS, Oni JA, Downing ND: Gadolinium enhanced MR assessment of proximal fragment vascularity in nonunions after scaphoid fracture: Does it predict the outcome of reconstructive surgery? *J Hand Surg Br* 2004;29:444-448.

55. Dailiana ZH, Zachos V, Varitimidis S, Papanagiotou P, Karantanas A, Malizos KN: Scaphoid nonunions treated with vascularized bone grafts: MRI assessment. *Eur J Radiol* 2004;50:217-224

CHAPTER 4

TREATMENT OF ACUTE SCAPHOID FRACTURES

MARCO RIZZO, MD
ALEXANDER Y. SHIN, MD
WILLIAM P. COONEY, MD

Scaphoid fractures are the most common carpal fracture and the second most common wrist fracture, following distal radius fractures. Although known as the most commonly fractured carpal bone in the wrist, the exact incidence remains unknown.[1-7] Scaphoid fractures typically occur in active, energetic adolescents and young adults, with a fourfold higher incidence in men compared with women.[4,6,7] Historically, scaphoid fractures were principally treated nonsurgically. However, our understanding of the consequences and disability that ensued from untreated acute scaphoid fractures, particularly displaced scaphoid fractures, began to be recognized. It became evident that displaced acute scaphoid fractures were prone to complications when left untreated, and complications such as nonunion, malunion, and progressive degenerative changes about the carpus occurred.

Both the recognition and treatment of acute scaphoid fractures have improved significantly over the past two decades. This is the result of improved training of physicians in evaluating a sprained wrist for fracture; improved imaging techniques, especially MRI; advances in surgical techniques as well as implants; and improved treatment regimens. Despite these advances, the treatment of the scaphoid fracture can be a challenge for both the surgeon and patient. This chapter reviews the current indications for surgical (versus nonsurgical) treatment of scaphoid fractures, the current recommendations for imaging, and the surgical techniques that provide for best outcomes in healing and functional clinical results.

DETERMINANTS OF TREATMENT

One role of classification of acute scaphoid fractures is to determine which fractures require surgical treatment and which can be effectively treated with immobilization; that is, identify which fractures are stable and which are unstable. The Herbert classification defines unstable scaphoid fractures as type B,[8] whereas the Mayo system defines an unstable fracture as one that has more than 1 mm of displacement or demonstrates carpal instability tendencies (scapholunate angle greater than 60°, radiolunate angle greater than 15°, or lateral intrascaphoid angle greater than 30°).[9] The first major determinant of treatment is the inherent stability of the scaphoid fracture. Stable fractures do not require manipulation to obtain a reduction, and typically include the Herbert type A and some B2 (nondisplaced complete waist fractures) fractures. As detailed later, we recommend nonsurgical treatment of most undisplaced scaphoid fractures and surgical treatment of displaced fractures.

The second determinant of treatment is fracture location. The average time to fracture union at the distal pole, scaphoid waist, and proximal pole has been estimated to be 6 weeks, 12 weeks, and 3 to 6 months, respectively. As a result of the prolonged need for immobilization of both displaced and nondisplaced proximal pole fractures and the propensity of these fractures to go on to nonunion with avascular changes of the proximal pole, surgical intervention has been advocated.[10]

The final determinant has nothing to do with the fracture or its configuration. These determinants of treatment are nonbiologic determinants and include considerations of socioeconomic factors (time-critical or sporting activities[11]) and psychiatric factors (inability to tolerate cast immobilization, noncompliance issues, patient follow-up expectations, etc).

Only after all three of the determinants are evaluated can a decision regarding surgical versus nonsurgical treatment be made.

CLOSED TREATMENT

Optimal treatment for nondisplaced or minimally displaced scaphoid fractures remains controversial. Prospective clinical studies comparing surgical intervention (open reduction and internal fixation) and nonsurgical treatments (closed reduction and cast immobilization) are necessary so that adequate comparisons can be made.[12] There is general agreement that the indication for closed treatment of scaphoid fractures is principally limited to stable, nondisplaced fractures of the distal third and waist of the scaphoid.[9,13] Nonsurgical methods of treatment for nondisplaced proximal pole fractures are more controversial, as discussed.[14,15] However, Dias and associates[16] questioned the role of surgical treatment of most scaphoid fractures and argued that cast immobilization is a time-proven, relatively complication-free method of treatment and that surgical treatment of acute scaphoid fractures should be reserved for those fractures that fail nonsurgical methods.

Early detection and treatment of scaphoid fractures is imperative to help ensure the best possible outcome. Multiple reports have demonstrated prolonged healing and nonunion with a delay in treatment.[17-20] This underscores the importance of high index of suspicion of potential fracture, early diagnosis (confirmed by routine or special imaging studies), and initiation of prompt treatment.

Multiple aspects of nonsurgical treatment of scaphoid fractures have been analyzed, including duration of casting, cast length,[21-26] whether the thumb should be immobilized,[25,27-31] wrist position,[31-36] and duration of casting.[9,37,38]

The position of immobilization of the wrist continues to been debated. O'Brien[35] felt that the ideal position of the wrist is flexion and radial deviation. Other data suggest that immobilization in flexion, although helpful in reducing the gap at the fracture site, likely leads to collapse.[31,32,36] Some surgeons argue that a position of flexion and radial deviation affords better approximation of the fracture fragments and reduces deforming forces across the wrist. However, King and colleagues[34] suggest that ulnar deviation and extension with the forearm supination is the best position for immobilization. Although no clear consensus has been reached,[39] most hand surgeons favor immobilization with the wrist in the neutral position.[40] The most important concept is that cast immobilization should be used not to maintain or reduce a scaphoid fracture; rather, it is used to prevent displacement of a stable, nondisplaced scaphoid fracture and maintain immobilization long enough for fracture healing. Any scaphoid fracture that requires reduction is inherently unstable, and surgical treatment should be considered.

Both below- and above-elbow immobilization have been recommended in the treatment of nondisplaced scaphoid fractures. There is some debate regarding the effect of forearm rotation on scaphoid fracture stability.[23,24,33,41,42] Kaneshiro and associates[33] noted approximately 4° of rotation and translation of simulated scaphoid fractures with forearm rotation. However, Falkenberg[23] found no significant fragment motion or rotation with supination or pronation in cadaveric wrists with simulated scaphoid fractures. More recently, McAdams and associates[41] performed a cadaver study using spiral CT reconstructions. The scaphoid was osteotomized, simulating a fracture. The investigators noted only an average of 0.2 mm motion at the fracture site using a below-the-elbow thumb spica cast. However, a clinical correlation is needed to determine whether this is a significant amount of motion to limit or reduce scaphoid fracture healing. Verdan[42] felt that shear forces occur across the scaphoid fracture site with pronation and supination of the wrist or forearm and recommended above-the-elbow immobilization. He felt that it neutralized the deforming force of the volar radiocarpal ligament.

Despite the disagreement on the necessity of above- versus below-elbow casting, clinical outcomes of both treatments are favorable.[19,22,24,25,43,44] Leslie and Dickson[38] evaluated 222 patients with scaphoid fractures treated in a short-arm thumb spica and reported a 95% union rate. Similarly, Stewart[25] reported union rates of 97% in military personnel treated with short-arm thumb spica casting. In contrast, Russe[44] documented a union rate of 97% in patients with scaphoid fractures treated initially with long-arm thumb spica immobilization.[44] Similar results were reported by Langhoff and Andersen[19]; their patients were treated initially with 4 weeks in a long-arm cast. Kuschner and associates[4] noted increased healing rate within a shorter period of time with long-arm cast immobilization.

Several studies directly compare the use of long and short-arm spica casting for nondisplaced scaphoid fractures.[21,24,43,45] Gellman and associates[24] prospectively evaluated 51 nondisplaced scaphoid fractures and found similar union rates. However, patients who wore a long-arm cast healed sooner (9.5 versus 12.7 weeks), and the nonunion rates were better (0 versus 2). Broome and associates[43] reiterated an improved healing rate, with 4 weeks of initial long-arm casting in a retrospective comparison. In contrast, Alho and Kankaanpaa[21] found no difference between the two groups, with a 92% union rate and 12 weeks until union. When deciding the best option, patient reliability is important. We recommend long-arm immobilization for noncompliant patients.[24,46] In compliant patients with stable scaphoid waist fractures, short-arm thumb spica cast immobilization until radiographic and clinical signs of healing are noted is recommended. In the midrange of patient compliance or if there is concern about any degree of fracture displacement, long-arm casting for the initial 4 to 6 weeks followed by conversion to short-arm casting should be considered.

SURGICAL TREATMENT OF UNSTABLE SCAPHOID FRACTURES

Displaced, comminuted, or unstable scaphoid fractures require surgical stabilization. Open reduction and internal fixation is the preferred technique.[26,36,47-50] Surgical techniques described for fixation of scaphoid fractures have included Kirschner wires (K-wires), screws, and staples. Both volar and dorsal approaches have been described. More recently, percutaneous techniques (pins and cannulated screws) have been reported, but most argue, at least for now, this is best performed in stable, minimally displaced, or nondisplaced fractures.[51-55] With more studies, the percutaneous technique may play a larger role in the surgical management of acute scaphoid fractures. The choice of fixation technique

depends on the location and configuration of the fracture, patient needs, functional concerns, and surgeon preference. We proceed in this section with a description of the volar and dorsal approaches for fracture reduction and internal fixation.

Volar Approach

The volar approach to scaphoid fractures was initially popularized by Russe[44] and generally is recommended for distal third and waist fractures.[56] Advantages of this approach include excellent visualization of the entire volar surface of the scaphoid, less likelihood of injury to the blood supply to the scaphoid, the ability to reduce scaphoid angulation deformity and carpal collapse, and adequate surface area of insertion of either a cancellous or corticocancellous bone graft, if needed. Disadvantages include capsular scarring and the resultant limited motion (especially extension), increased risk of carpal instability related to dissection, and failure to fully repair the volar carpal ligaments.[10,57] Another reported problem with this approach is the potential for scaphotrapezial trapezoid arthrosis secondary to insertion of a distal-to-proximal scaphoid screw. However, multiple reports describe excellent healing rates using the volar approach for either acute displaced scaphoid fractures or scaphoid nonunions.[8,10,58-60]

The surgical approach uses the interval between the flexor carpi radialis and the radial artery (**Figure 1**). The superficial branch of the radial artery is commonly ligated to facilitate visualization of the scaphoid. The volar capsule and volar radiocarpal ligaments (the radioscaphocapitate and long radiolunate ligaments) are divided and suture tagged for later repair. The exposure allows for direct visualization of the fracture site. In some cases, only a very faint fracture line is visible and in others a clear displacement is evident. If substantial comminution is present, then cancellous bone grafting may be necessary to facilitate anatomic reduction and healing. The reduction is facilitated and maintained with a provisional K-wire. Care is taken to ensure that the K-wire corrects both dorsal palmar and any rotational malalignment of the scaphoid. In addition, the provisional wire should not be in a position to interfere with the cannulated compression screw. When the scaphoid screw is inserted from distal to proximal (retrograde approach), it may be necessary to take down the lateral

FIGURE 1

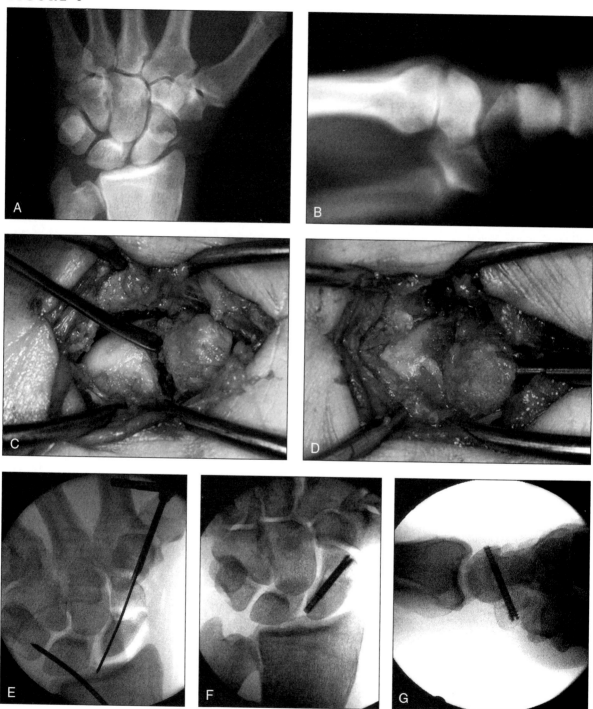

The volar approach for surgical treatment of scaphoid fractures. PA **(A)** and lateral **(B)** radiographs showing the fracture. **C,** Exposure of the fracture site through the volar approach. **D,** The compression variable pitch screw has been placed. Fluoroscopic images showing placement of the guide pin **(E)**, and final screw placement **(F and G)**.

volar lip of the scaphotrapezial joint to achieve the appropriate starting point for the screw. The Herbert screw system uses compression jigs (Heung jig) to maintain and compress the reduction while screw is being placed. Following placement of the guide pin, the screw length is calculated with a depth gauge. The guide pin is then overdrilled, and the screw is inserted. Radiographic assistance is helpful in evaluating wire and screw placements. Placing the screw in the central third of the scaphoid has been shown to decrease time to union.[61]

Dorsal Radial Approach

The dorsal radial approach to scaphoid fractures was initially described by McLaughlin[62] and is now recommended by hand surgeons for limited open or percutaneous fixation of proximal pole scaphoid fractures. The advantage of this approach is that improved fixation of the proximal pole fractures can be achieved. And with the increase control of the proximal and middle thirds of the scaphoid, many authors preferred this approach for proximal pole and scaphoid waist fractures.[10,63] Also, visualization of the important scapholunate ligament with surgical repair can be performed, if necessary. Finally, this approach spares the important volar supporting extrinsic ligaments. The disadvantages of this approach include difficulty in visualizing the entire scaphoid and more difficult intraoperative imaging. Despite the theoretically increased risk of blood supply disruption, there have been no incidences of osteonecrosis of the scaphoid reported.[10,64-66] Multiple reports of achieving successful union of scaphoid fractures through a dorsal approach have been published.[10,64,65]

The dorsal approach is performed through a longitudinal or transverse incision centered over Lister's tubercle (**Figure 2**). Care is taken to identify and protect branches of the dorsal sensory branch of the radial nerve. The extensor retinaculum is divided between the third and fourth compartments, and the extensor pollicis longus is removed from within the retinaculum and safely retracted. Care is taken to protect the dorsal radial blood vessels to the scaphoid, notably the branch off of the radial artery to the dorsal ridge and entering into the waist of the scaphoid. To visualize proximal pole fractures, the wrist must be flexed. Occasionally a portion of the dorsal lip of the radius must be removed with a rongeur to facilitate visualization. The fracture

is then reduced and provisional fixation obtained with a K-wire. Again, care must be taken to avoid placing the wire in the proposed line of the screw. Radiography assists in confirming both adequate reduction and pin placement. The guidewire is then placed and proposed screw length measured with a depth gauge. With a cannulated screw system, the scaphoid is first drilled (self-drilling, self-tapping screw) and then the screw is inserted. With some cannulated screw systems, compression of the scaphoid may occur and there is potential for collapse; it is therefore recommended to subtract 2 mm from the measured screw length. With a noncannulated screw system, the central K-wire is again inserted (with a second K-wire to control rotational stresses), the depth or length of the K-wire (and subsequent screw is measured and confirmed by C-arm imaging), the drill or a larger K-wire inserted down the same track as the original K-wire, and then the noncannulated screw inserted.

Postoperative treatment after open reduction and fixation of scaphoid fractures is similar for either approach. Patients are placed in thumb spica immobilization initially. Generally, a short-arm cast is recommended for 6 to 8 weeks or until radiographic union is achieved after open reduction and fixation of unstable scaphoid fractures. CT can be helpful in assessing healing.[10] Radiographic union should occur by 7 to 8 weeks; however, proximal pole fractures may take 12 weeks or longer to show evidence of radiographic healing .

PERCUTANEOUS TECHNIQUES FOR STABLE SCAPHOID FRACTURES

Over the past decade, there has been an increased interest in minimally invasive surgical techniques for treatment of scaphoid fractures. Rigid internal fixation of scaphoid fractures via percutaneous approaches have the benefit of minimal soft-tissue injury and a reported increased rate of fracture healing and subsequently earlier return to work and/or sports.[51,53,54,67-69] Percutaneous approaches have been described for dorsal and volar fixation techniques.[51,53,54,67-69] The indications, contraindications, techniques, rehabilitation, complications, and results of treatment for volar percutaneous technique are discussed herein.

FIGURE 2

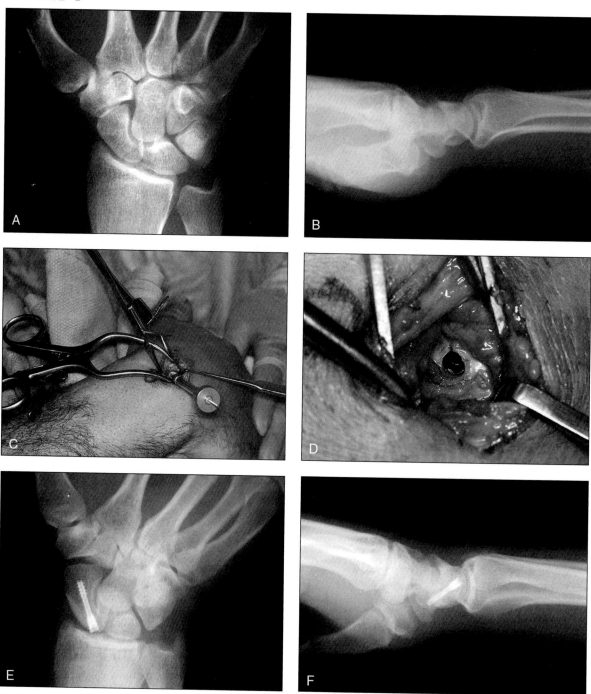

The dorsal approach for surgical treatment of scaphoid fractures. PA **(A)** and lateral **(B)** radiographs show a proximal pole fracture. A transverse incision was used in this case. After placement of the guidewire, the depth was measured **(C)**. Fluoroscopy helps to confirm adequate placement of the K-wire. The scaphoid is drilled **(D)**, and screws are inserted. Postoperative PA **(E)** and lateral **(F)** radiographs demonstrate the anatomic reduction.

In an attempt to decrease the time of fracture immobilization with the subsequent wrist stiffness, loss of strength, and loss of economic productivity or athletic endeavors, several authors have reported on acute screw percutaneous fixation techniques for scaphoid fractures.[8,51,53,54,67-76] Although open exposure of the scaphoid allows for better fracture alignment and perhaps more accurate fixation, it does require division of the very important volar radiocarpal ligaments or dorsal capsular structures. A percutaneously placed compression screw, however, avoids these potential pitfalls, and allow for earlier motion and rehabilitation. In 1970, Streli[68] first reported the technique of percutaneous screw fixation for fractures of the scaphoid. In 1991, Wozasek and Moser[69] retrospectively evaluated the results of the volar percutaneous screw fixation technique and demonstrated an 89% healing rate of percutaneous screw fixation of acute scaphoid fracture healing in 146 patients after an average of 4.2 months. These authors concluded that good results could be anticipated with percutaneous screw fixation. Inoue and Shinonoya[53] retrospectively reported on 40 patients treated with Wozasek and Moser's technique, and demonstrated fracture union at 6 weeks compared with a cohort of fractures treated nonsurgically, which averaged 9.7 weeks to union; they recommended percutaneous fixation because it allowed for earlier return to work and 100% union rate.

The goals of surgery include early motion and return to activity while ensuring a high union rate and avoiding the problems associated with prolonged immobilization. The volar percutaneous screw fixation technique is indicated primarily for minimally and nondisplaced scaphoid waist fractures. Displacement of more than 1 mm and fracture comminution are indications for open reduction or an arthroscopically assisted method to obtain anatomic alignment. However, the technique can be successfully applied to displaced fractures that can be easily reduced by ulnar deviation and wrist extension. Fracture pattern and location is of critical importance; a transverse waist fracture is ideally suited to stable fixation with a screw placed from the volar distal direction. Conversely, this technique is contraindicated in proximal pole and oblique fractures because the screw cannot perpendicularly cross the fracture line and obtain adequate compression and purchase. Distal pole fractures can present the same

technical difficulties. These are considered relative contraindications to the technique and are subject to patient and surgeon preferences.

Another relative contraindication is the occult scaphoid fracture; when the patient has a mechanism and examination consistent with fracture but negative radiographic studies. After 2 weeks of immobilization, the fracture line becomes visible where resorption and new bony trabeculation have occurred. Although this technique could be used, we often opt for nonsurgical management in these patients because the healing process has already begun when the definitive diagnosis is made.

Although percutaneous screw fixation is highly successful, both the surgeon and patient must be aware that if the fracture is further displaced or inadequately reduced intraoperatively, then open reduction is required. As such, a thorough preoperative discussion regarding the potential for displacement of a nondisplaced fracture requiring formal open reduction and internal fixation is requisite.

Volar Percutaneous Scaphoid Screw Fixation

Once anesthetized with a general or regional anesthetic, the patient is placed on the operating table in the supine position with the arm abducted on a radiolucent arm board (**Figure 3**). Although a tourniquet is placed on the brachium, it is not routinely used. Placement of the fluoroscopy unit depends on the handedness of the surgeon. A right-handed surgeon operating on a right scaphoid feels most comfortable placing the guide wires seated superiorly to the arm, with the image intensifier coming from inferiorly. Two rolled towels are used under the supinated wrist to allow for adequate dorsiflexion.

The guidewire for the cannulated screw system is placed through the volar scaphoid tuberosity, directed proximally, dorsally, and ulnarly with the wrist hyperextended. Image intensification is used in multiple planes to ensure that the wire is placed along the longitudinal axis of the scaphoid and across the fracture site. Next, a second guidewire is placed parallel to the first guidewire for antirotation control. This wire must cross the fracture and be far enough away from the initial guidewire as not to interfere with the drill or screw. Dorsiflexion of the wrist assists in translating the trapezium out of the path of the wire, making placement easier and

FIGURE 3

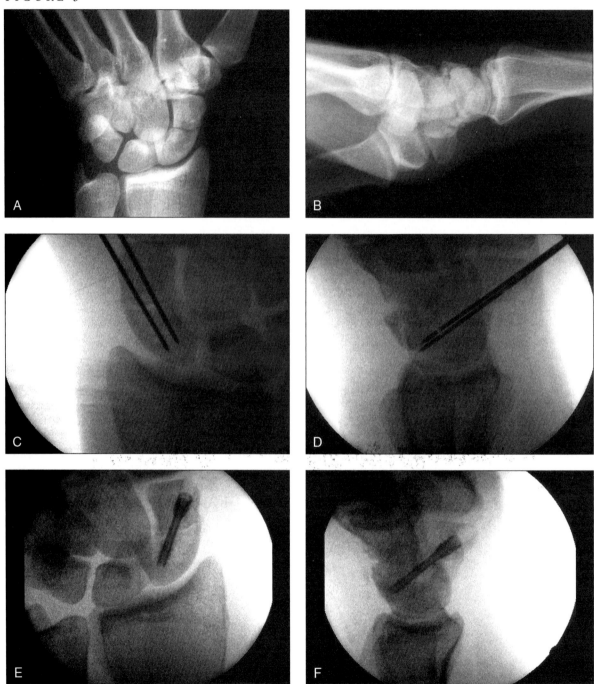

The volar technique for surgical treatment of scaphoid fractures. PA **(A)** and lateral **(B)** radiographs show a midscaphoid fracture. Fluoroscopic images showing placement of the first guide pin, a derotational second K-wire **(C)**, and confirmation of adequate positioning **(D)**. The guide pins are then drilled, and the appropriate length screw is inserted. Postoperative fluoroscopic PA **(E)** and lateral **(F)** images show anatomic alignment and good screw placement.

avoiding disrupting the scaphotrapeziotrapezoid joint. It is also important to understand that the position of the screw within the scaphoid is not along the long axis of the scaphoid but is slightly diagonal to it.

Screw length can be measured with the measuring device available in the screw set, or alternatively indirectly with a second guide pin. It is important to subtract 1 to 2 mm from the measured length of the guidewire; the screw should be completely buried within the scaphoid, and there should be an allowance for minor scaphoid collapse. We have found little variation in screw length: a 20.0-mm screw suffices in almost all cases, with a 17.5- or 22.5-mm screw being used in the remainder of cases.

A 3-mm incision is made around the guide pin to allow drill and screw passage. The scaphoid is then hand drilled with the graduated cannulated drill, with the depth monitored by fluoroscopy. The cannulated screw is placed with fluoroscopic guidance to judge fracture reduction and screw position. Final fluoroscopic images are obtained, as well as a live view of the reduction. The antirotation guidewire is removed, the wound irrigated and closed with a nylon suture. A well-padded, short-arm thumb spica splint is applied.

When choosing a cannulated screw, it is important that the guidewire be at least 1 mm in diameter. Additionally, it is important to know the nuances of the screw system that is chosen.

Dorsal Percutaneous Screw Fixation

Several methods of dorsal percutaneous fixation of scaphoid fractures have been described, each of which demands precise placement of the guidewire down the central anatomic axis of the scaphoid. By pronating, flexing, and ulnarly deviating the wrist, the scaphoid can be viewed with fluoroscopy as a cylinder (**Figure 4**). A guidewire that is introduced down the center of this cylinder is placed along the central anatomic axis of the scaphoid.[54,55] Alternatively, the guidewire can be placed on the proximal aspect of the scaphoid side of the scapholunate ligament while the wrist is flexed. Advancing the wire parallel to the extensor pollicis longus tendon allows the wire to be advanced along the central anatomic axis (**Figure 5**). With both of these methods of introducing the guidewire, the wire is advanced across the scaphoid fracture site. The pin is then advanced

through the volar skin and withdrawn until the radio-carpal joint can be extended without being blocked by the guidewire. Fluoroscopy is then used to confirm the reduction and guide wire placement. If the fracture is displaced, the guidewire is further advanced to be in only the distal portion of the scaphoid, and an adequate reduction usually can be accomplished with positioning of the wrist. Alternatively, percutaneous 0.045- to 0.062-inch K-wires can be used as joysticks to align the fracture. The guidewire is then advanced retrograde, leaving it exposed volarly to prevent accidental removal with reaming. Next, a second guidewire is placed parallel to the first guide wire for antirotation control. This wire must cross the fracture and be far enough away from the initial guidewire as not to interfere with the drill or screw.

A 3-mm incision is made around the guide pin to allow drill and screw passage. The scaphoid is then drilled with the graduated cannulated drill, with the depth monitored by fluoroscopy. The scaphoid is drilled within 2 mm of the distal cortex, and screw length can be measured directly off of the markings on the scaphoid drill (or reamer). Alternatively, screw length can be obtained from preoperative radiographs of the uninjured scaphoid, or a third guidewire laid over the skin and clamped after confirming with fluoroscopy can be measured.

The cannulated screw is placed with fluoroscopic guidance to judge fracture reduction and screw position. The antirotation guidewire is removed, and final fluoroscopic images are obtained, as well as a live view of the reduction.

Complications

This is a safe surgical procedure, but there are some potential pitfalls. One is the possibility of displacing the fracture, which usually is caused by inaccurate placement of the guidewire and a drill or screw crossing the fracture at an oblique angle. Displacement is especially likely to occur in proximal pole or oblique fractures, again emphasizing the need for proper patient selection. The patient must give informed consent for and the surgeon prepared to perform an open reduction in such a case. Placing a screw with inadequate purchase or in a malreduced fracture can have potentially disastrous consequences. Screws placed into the capitate rather than proximal scaphoid, cannulated screws that are too long

FIGURE 4

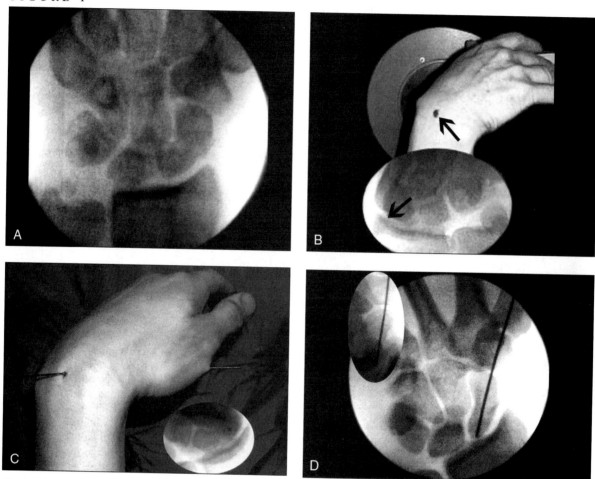

The dorsal approach for percutaneous stabilization of scaphoid fractures (Slade technique). **A,** PA fluoroscopic image of the wrist shows the central axis of the scaphoid. **B,** The wrist is then flexed and pronated until the scaphoid cylinder appears as a circle. The central axis of the scaphoid is now in the imaging beam, at the center of the scaphoid circle. The arrow in the radiograph and the dot on the photograph of the dorsal part of the wrist show the central axis of the scaphoid and the position and direction of the guidewire. **C,** The wrist is then extended, and minifluoroscopy is used to confirm the position of the guidewire along the central axis of the scaphoid, as well as the quality of the fracture reduction. **D,** Fluoroscopy confirms anatomic reduction of the following screw placement. (Reproduced with permission from Slade JF, Gutow AP, Geissler WB: Percutaneous internal fixation of scaphoid fractures via an arthroscopically assisted dorsal approach. *J Bone Joint Surg Am* 2002;84(suppl 2):21-36.)

have come out through the proximal scaphoid, and scaphoid fixation in a malreduced position have all been reported. For this reason alone, surgeon experience in the technique, patient and fracture selection, and the consent and need to change techniques if the percutaneous procedure proves difficult are critical requirements for this technique.

One problem unique to this technique is that of

obtaining accurate drill depth. Overdrilling can lead to a loose screw with poor purchase; underdrilling could potentially split the bone when the screw is placed and also may lead to distraction across the fracture fragments. This problem can be avoided by drilling under fluoroscopic guidance and placing the drill and screw at the same depth. Failure to completely bury the head of the screw within the scaphoid can lead to scapho-

FIGURE 5

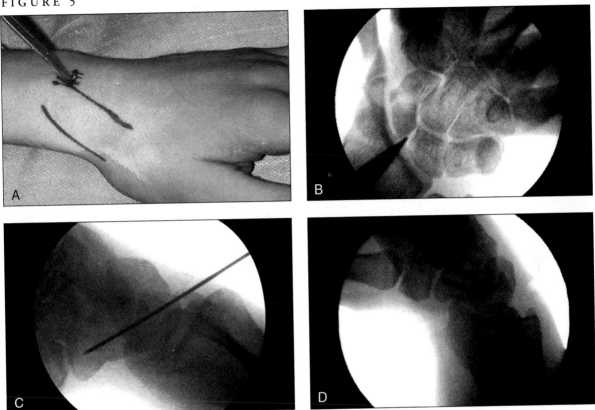

The dorsal approach for percutaneous stabilization of scaphoid fractures (non-Slade technique). **A,** Markings on the skin show depict the path of the scaphoid, and the incision site is just ulnar to the ulnar line proximally. **B,** PA radiograph shows the appropriate starting point. **C,** Insertion of the K-wire guide pin in line with the scaphoid. **D,** Lateral fluoroscopic image following placement of a cannulated compression screw. (Courtesy of Klaus Werber, Germany.)

trapeziotrapezoid arthrosis distally and to radioscaphoid arthritis proximally, and may require subsequent screw removal. This complication can be avoided by selecting a screw length approximately 1 to 2 mm shorter than that actually measured.

Although the radial artery is a concern in surgical treatment of scaphoid fractures, it is in no danger if surgical techniques are properly performed. The radial artery branches proximal to the scaphoid, and there are no vascular or neural structures overlying the tuberosity. Anatomic studies have demonstrated the guidewire placed into the scaphoid through the tuberosity to be 14 mm from the radial artery, 19 mm from the superficial branch of the radial nerve, and 5 mm from the superficial branch of the radial artery.[77] The prudent surgeon must be knowledgeable of the anatomy, but as long as the guidewires are placed into the scaphoid under fluoroscopic guidance and care is taken to avoid making errant passes into soft tissue, the risk of damage to the radial artery is minimal.

Postoperative Rehabilitation

Digital range of motion and edema control are initiated on postoperative day 1. The hand is kept in a surgical dressing with a volar plaster splint for 10 days, at which time the splint and sutures are removed. The patient is then placed into a molded orthoplast short-arm thumb spica splint for 3 weeks. During this time, the splint is removed for gentle wrist motion and hygiene. Radiographic and clinical union are typically achieved at 6 to 7 weeks. The splint is discontinued, and all previous activities are resumed as tolerated.

Results

Nonsurgical treatment of most nondisplaced scaphoid fractures usually results in good to excellent outcomes in most patients. Cast immobilization of scaphoid fractures has resulted in fracture union in approximately 95% of scaphoid waist fractures.[78] Other studies of cast immobilization, (both long- and short-arm casts) are efficient in producing union of nondisplaced and minimally displaced scaphoid fractures. The recent application of cannulated screws has produced similar union rates and at the same time decreased the time for immobilization of the wrist. Some authors are concerned about the increased used of screw fixation when nonsurgical means have been demonstrated to be successful.

Screw fixation of displaced scaphoid fractures also has demonstrated good to excellent results. Filan and Herbert[59] reviewed their experience with a compression screw and reported an 85% to 90% union rate for various types of acute fractures. Rettig and associates[79] reviewed the Mayo experience with displaced scaphoid fractures, all of which were treated by open reduction and internal fixation with compression screws. Complete fracture union with near-normal motion and grip strength was reported in 93% of patients.

The results of percutaneous screw fixation of scaphoid fractures have been promising. Wozasek and Moser[69] reported an 89% healing rate with this technique in a variety of scaphoid fracture types, with an average healing time of 4.2 months. Inoue and Shinonoya[53] demonstrated that percutaneous screw fixation had a shorter time to union compared with a cohort of scaphoid fractures treated nonsurgically. The average time to union in the percutaneous screw fixation cohort was 6 weeks compared with 9.7 weeks for fractures treated nonsurgically, with earlier return to work for the percutaneous fixation cohort. In a prospective randomized study of nondisplaced scaphoid waist fractures treated with percutaneous screw fixation versus cast immobilization, Bond and associates[51] demonstrated statistically significant differences in time to union and return to work. This series showed that fracture healing in patients who underwent percutaneous screw fixation averaged 7.1 weeks compared with 11.6 weeks for cast immobilization. Similarly, patients who had percutaneous screw fixation returned to work at an average of 8.2 weeks, versus 15.3 weeks for cast immobilization. There were no nonunions, and only one patient had a prominent painful screw that required subsequent removal. Another prospective randomized study came to different conclusions. Adolfsson and associates[80] prospectively randomized 53 patients to a percutaneous volar screw fixation or cast immobilization. Radiographs were obtained at 10 and 16 weeks, and the patients who underwent screw fixation were allowed to return to work at 6 weeks, regardless of union status. They concluded that there were no statistical differences between groups with respect to time to union or rate of union, but patients who underwent surgery had better range of motion with earlier return to work.

ARTHROSCOPICALLY ASSISTED REDUCTION

Arthroscopically assisted fixation of scaphoid fractures has been lauded as an improved means of assessing adequate reduction of the scaphoid. It can be done in association with percutaneous fixation, and the technique has the additional advantage of diagnosing associated and/or additional soft-tissue injuries.[54,76,81] Shih and colleagues[81] evaluated 15 scaphoid fractures treated percutaneously with arthroscopic assistance. All of the fractures healed; complications included triangular fibrocartilage complex tears, lunotriquetral and partial scapholunate ligament injuries, extrinsic (radioscaphocapitate, long radiolunate) ligament injuries, and chondral injuries. Many of these required surgical intervention. There were 11 excellent and 4 good results. A separate review of 16 fractures was reported using an arthroscopically assisted dorsal percutaneous technique.[54] Despite the fact that six fractures were treated late (>1 month after injury), all healed at an average of 12 weeks. The authors reported no complications in their series.

The technique initially involves arthroscopy to visualize the fracture fragments and clean out fracture hematoma. The remaining aspects of both the radio- and midcarpal joints are inspected to evaluate for associated injuries. Typical portals are used, including the 3-

4, 4-5, and 6R (or U) portals in the radiocarpal joints. In addition, the midcarpal, radial, and ulnar portals are used (typically providing optimal views for seeing the fracture and subsequent reduction). The scaphoid fracture is then reduced under direct visualization. This can be performed with K-wires and confirmed with fluoroscopy. If necessary, K-wires can be placed into each fragment and manipulated to facilitate reduction. Following reduction, screw placement is similar to the volar and dorsal percutaneous techniques. Compression and reduction maintenance can be visualized arthroscopically. Postoperative care and rehabilitation are similar to the percutaneous technique.

CONCLUSION

The scaphoid is a key element in the carpal functions of the wrist. It is quite susceptible to injury and fracture, and when injured requires prompt diagnosis, with a specific and defined treatment plan. Early diagnosis and appropriate treatment allows union in most patients and avoids the sequelae of the scaphoid fracture nonunion. A thorough understanding of the anatomy, pathomechanics of the wrist, and treatment options is necessary in planning the optimal treatment plan for patients with scaphoid nonunions.

REFERENCES

1. Borgeskov S, Christiansen B, Kjaer A, Balslev I: Fractures of the carpal bones. *Acta Orthop Scand* 1966;37:276-287.

2. Fisk GR: Carpal instability and the fractured scaphoid. *Ann R Coll Surg Engl* 1970;46:63-76.

3. Kozin SH: Incidence, mechanism, and natural history of scaphoid fractures. *Hand Clin* 2001;17:515-524.

4. Kuschner SH, Lane CS, Brien WW, Gellman H: Scaphoid fractures and scaphoid nonunion: Diagnosis and treatment. *Orthop Rev* 1994;23:861-871.

5. London PS: The broken scaphoid bone: The case against pessimism. *J Bone Joint Surg Br* 1961;43:237-244

6. Osterman AL, Mikulics M: Scaphoid nonunion. *Hand Clin* 1988;4:437-455.

7. Trumble TE, Salas P, Barthel T, Robert KQ III: Management of scaphoid nonunions. *J Am Acad Orthop Surg* 2003;11:380-391.

8. Herbert TJ, Fisher WE: Management of the fractured scaphoid using a new bone screw. *J Bone Joint Surg Br* 1984;66:114-123.

9. Cooney WP, Dobyns JH, Linscheid RL: Fractures of the scaphoid: A rational approach to management. *Clin Orthop* 1980;149:90-97.

10. Rettig ME, Raskin KB: Retrograde compression screw fixation of acute proximal pole scaphoid fractures. *J Hand Surg Am* 1999;24:1206-1210.

11. Geissler WB: Carpal fractures in athletes. *Clin Sports Med* 2001;20:167-188.

12. Bhandari M, Hanson BP: Acute nondisplaced fractures of the scaphoid. *J Orthop Trauma* 2004;18:253-255.

13. Terkelsen CJ, Jepsen JM: Treatment of scaphoid fractures with a removable cast. *Acta Orthop Scand* 1988;59:452-453.

14. Alnot JY, Bellan N, Oberlin C, De Cheveigne C: Fractures and nonunions of the proximal pole of the carpal scaphoid bone: Internal fixation by a proximal to distal screw. *Ann Chir Main* 1988;7:101-108.

15. Rehbein F, Düben W: Zur konservativen behandlung des veralteten kahnbeinbruches und der kahnbein-pseudarthrose. *Arch Orthop Unfall Chir* 1952;45:67-77.

16. Dias JJ, Wildin CJ, Bhowal B, Thompson JR: Should acute scaphoid fractures be fixed? A randomized controlled trial. *J Bone Joint Surg Am* 2005;87:2160-2168.

17. Dickison JC, Shannon JG: Fractures of the carpal scaphoid in the Canadian Army. *Surg Gynecol Obstet* 1944;79:225.

18. Eddeland A, Eiken O, Hellgren E, Ohlsson NM: Fractures of the scaphoid. *Scand J Plast Reconstr Surg* 1975;9:234-239.

19. Langhoff O, Andersen JL: Consequences of late immobilization of scaphoid fractures. *J Hand Surg Br* 1988;13:77-79.

20. Mack GR, Wilckens JH, McPherson SA: Subacute scaphoid fractures: A closer look at closed treatment. *Am J Sports Med* 1998;26:56-58

21. Alho A, Kankaanpaa U: Management of fractured scaphoid bone: A prospective study of 100 fractures. *Acta Orthop Scand* 1975;46:737-743.

22. Dickson RA, Leslie IJ: Conservative treatment of the fractured scaphoid, in Razemon JP, Fisk GR (eds): *The Wrist*. Edinburgh, Churchill Livingstone, 1988, p 80.

23. Falkenberg P: An experimental study of instability during supination and pronation of the fractured scaphoid. *J Hand Surg Br* 1985;10:211-213.

24. Gellman H, Caputo RJ, Carter V, Aboulafia A, McKay M: Comparison of short and long thumb-spica casts for non-displaced fractures of the carpal scaphoid. *J Bone Joint Surg Am* 1990;72:309-310.

25. Stewart MJ: Fractures of the carpal navicular (scaphoid): A report of 436 cases. *J Bone Joint Surg Am* 1954;36:998-1006.

26. Verdan C, Narakas A: Fractures and pseudarthrosis of the scaphoid. *Surg Clin North Am* 1968;48:1083-1095.

27. Burge P: Closed cast treatment of scaphoid fractures. *Hand Clin* 2001;17:541-552.

28. Clay NR, Dias JJ, Costigan PS, Gregg PJ, Barton NJ: Need the thumb be immobilized in scaphoid fractures: A randomized prospective trial. *J Bone Joint Surg Br* 1991;73:828-832.

29. Herbert TJ: *The Fractured Scaphoid.* St. Louis, MO, Quality Medical Publishing, 1990.

30. Soto-Hall R, Haldeman KO: The conservative and operative treatment of fractures of the carpal scaphoid (navicular). *J Bone Joint Surg* 1941;23:841.

31. Weber ER, Chao EYS: An experimental approach to the mechanism of scaphoid waist fractures. *J Hand Surg Am* 1978;3:142-148.

32. Hambidge JE, Desai VV, Schranz PJ, Compson JP, Davis TR, Barton NJ: Acute fractures of the scaphoid: Treatment by cast immobilization with the wrist in flexion or extension? *J Bone Joint Surg Br* 1999;81:91-102.

33. Kaneshiro SA, Failla JM, Tashman S: Scaphoid fracture displacement with forearm rotation in a short-arm thumb spica cast. *J Hand Surg Am* 1999;24:984-991

34. King RJ, Mackenney RP, Elnur S: Suggested method for closed treatment of fractures of the carpal scaphoid: Hypothesis supported by dissection and clinical practice. *J R Soc Med* 1982;75:860-867.

35. O'Brien E: *Acute Fractures and Dislocations of the Carpus.* Philadelphia, PA, WB Saunders, 1988.

36. Weber ER: Biomechanical implications of scaphoid waist fractures. *Clin Orthop* 1980;149:83-89

37. Böhler L (ed): *Técnica del Tratamiento de las Fracturas,* ed 3 [translated from German, vol. 1, ed 7]. Barcelona, Editorial Labor SA, 1954.

38. Leslie IJ, Dickson RA: The fractured carpal scaphoid: Natural history and factors influencing outcome. *J Bone Joint Surg Br* 1981;63:225-230.

39. Smith DK, Cooney WP III, An KN, Linscheid RL, Chao EYS: The effects of simulated unstable scaphoid frac-tures on carpal motion. *J Hand Surg Am* 1989;14:283-291.

40. Jupiter JB, Shin AY, Trumble TE, Fernandez DL: Trau-matic and reconstructive problems of the scaphoid. *Instr Course Lect* 2001;50:105-122.

41. McAdams TR, Spisak S, Beaulieu CF, Ladd AL: The effect of pronation and supination on the minimally displaced scaphoid fracture. *Clin Orthop Relat Res* 2003;411:255-259.

42. Verdan C: Le role du ligament anterieur radiocarpien dans les fractures du scaphoide: Deductions therapeu-tiques [The role of anterior radiocarpal ligament in fractures of the scaphoid carpus; therapeutic deduc-tions]. *Z Unfallmed Berufskr* 1954;47:294-297.

43. Broome A, Cedell CA, Colleen S: High plaster immo-bilisation for fracture of the carpal scaphoid bone. *Acta Chir Scand* 1964;128:42-44.

44. Russe O: Fracture of the carpal navicular: Diagnosis, non-operative treatment and operative treatment. *J Bone Joint Surg Am* 1960;42:759-768

45. Goldman S, Lipscomb PR, Taylor WF: Immobilization for acute carpal scaphoid fractures. *Surg Gynecol Obstet* 1969;129:281-284.

46. Krasin E, Goldwirth M, Gold A, Goodwin DR: Review of the current methods in the diagnosis and treatment of scaphoid fractures. *Postgrad Med J* 2001;77:235-237.

47. Cugola L, Testoni R: Bone fixation with shape memory staples, in Saffar P, Amadio P, Foucher G (eds): *Current Practice in Hand Surgery.* London, Martin Dunitz, 1997, p 84.

48. Maudsley RH, Chen SC: Screw fixation in the manage-ment of the fractured carpal scaphoid. *J Bone Joint Surg Br* 1972;54:432-441.

49. McLaughlin HL, Parkes JC II: Fracture of the carpal navicular (scaphoid) bone: Gradations in therapy based upon pathology. *J Trauma* 1969;9:311-319.

50. Yang PJ, Zhang YF, Ge MZ, Cai TD, Tao JC, Yang HP: Internal fixation with Ni-Tl shape memory alloy com-pressive staples in orthopedic surgery: A review of 51 cases. *Chin Med J* 1987;100:712-719

51. Bond CD, Shin AY, McBride MT, Dao KD: Percuta-neous screw fixation or cast immobilization for nondis-placed scaphoid fractures. *J Bone Joint Surg Am* 2001;83:483-488.

52. Haddad FS, Goddard NJ: Acute percutaneous scaphoid fixation: A pilot study. *J Bone Joint Surg Br* 1998;80:95-99.

53. Inoue G, Shinonoya K: Herbert screw fixation by limited access for acute fractures of the scaphoid. *J Bone Joint Surg Br* 1997;79:418-421.

54. Slade JF III, Grauer JN, Mahoney JD: Arthroscopic reduction and percutaneous fixation of scaphoid fractures with a novel dorsal technique. *Orthop Clin North Am* 2001;32:247-261.

55. Slade JF, Gutow AP, Geissler WB: Percutaneous internal fixation of scaphoid fractures via an arthroscopically assisted dorsal approach. *J Bone Joint Surg Am* 2002;84(suppl 2):21-36.

56. Cooney WP III: Scaphoid fractures: current treatments and techniques. *Instr Course Lect* 2003;52:197-208.

57. Garcia-Elias M, Vall A, Salo JM, Lluch AL: Carpal alignment after different surgical approaches to the scaphoid: A comparative study. *J Hand Surg Am* 1988;13:604-612.

58. Bunker TD, McNamee PB, Scott TD: The Herbert screw for scaphoid fractures: A multicentre study. *J Bone Joint Surg Br* 1987;69:631-634.

59. Filan SL, Herbert TJ: Herbert screw fixation of scaphoid fractures. *J Bone Joint Surg Br* 1996;78:519-529.

60. Trumble TE, Gilbert M, Murray LW, Smith J: Displaced scaphoid fractures treated with open reduction and internal fixation with a cannulated screw. *J Bone Joint Surg Am* 2000;82:633-641.

61. Trumble TE, Clarke T, Kreder HJ: Non-union of the scaphoid: Treatment with cannulated screws compared with treatment with Herbert screws. *J Bone Joint Surg Am* 1996;78:1829-1837

62. McLaughlin HL: Fracture of the carpal navicular (scaphoid) bone: Some observations based on treatment by open reduction and internal fixation. *J Bone Joint Surg Am* 1954;36:765-774.

63. Trumble T, Nyland W: Scaphoid nonunions: Pitfalls and pearls. *Hand Clin* 2001;17:611-624.

64. DeMaagd RL, Engber WD: Retrograde Herbert screw fixation for treatment of proximal pole scaphoid nonunions. *J Hand Surg Am* 1989;14:996-1003.

65. dos Reis FB, Koeberle G, Leite NM, Katchburian MV: Internal fixation of scaphoid injuries using the Herbert screw through a dorsal approach. *J Hand Surg Am* 1993;18:792-797.

66. Watson HK, Pitta EC, Ashmead IV D, Makhlouf MV, Kauer J: Dorsal approach to scaphoid nonunion. *J Hand Surg Am* 1993;18:359-365.

67. Haddad FS, Goddard NJ: Acute percutaneous scaphoid fixation using a cannulated screw. *Ann Chir Main* 1998;17:119-126.

68. Streli R: Perkutane Vershraubung des Handkahnbeines mit Bohrdrahtkompressionschraube. *Zentralbl Chir* 1970;95:1060-1078.

69. Wozasek GE, Moser KD: Percutaneous screw fixation for fractures of the scaphoid [published erratum appears in *J Bone Joint Surg Br* 1991 May;73:524]. *J Bone Joint Surg Br* 1991;73:138-142.

70. Huene DR: Primary internal fixation of carpal navicular fractures in the athlete. *Am J Sports Med* 1979;7:175-177.

71. Kozin SH: Internal fixation of scaphoid fractures. *Hand Clin* 1997;13:573-586.

72. O'Brien L, Herbert TJ: Internal fixation of acute scaphoid fractures: A new approach to treatment. *Aust N Z J Surg* 1985;55:387-389.

73. Rettig AC: Fractures in the hand in athletes. *Instr Course Lect* 1998;47:187-190.

74. Rettig AC, Kollias SC: Internal fixation of acute stable scaphoid fractures in the athlete. *Am J Sports Med* 1996;24:182-186.

75. Rettig AC, Weidenbener EJ, Gloyeske R: Alternative management of midthird scaphoid fractures in the athlete. *Am J Sports Med* 1994;22:711-714.

76. Whipple TL: Stabilization of the fractured scaphoid under arthroscopic control. *Orthop Clin North Am* 1995;26:749-754.

77. Kamineni S, Lavy CB: Percutaneous fixation of scaphoid fractures: An anatomic study. *J Hand Surg Br* 1999;24:85-88.

78. Leslie IJ, Dickson RA: The fractured carpal scaphoid: Natural history and factors influencing outcome *J Bone Joint Surg Br* 1981;63:225-230.

79. Rettig ME, Kozin SH, Cooney WP: Open reduction and internal fixation of acute displaced scaphoid waist fractures. *J Hand Surg Am* 2001;26:271-276.

80. Adolfsson L, Lindau T, Arner M: Acutrak screw fixation versus cast immobilization for undisplaced scaphoid waist fractures. *J Hand Surg Br* 2001;26:192-195.

81. Shih JT, Lee HM, Hou YT, Tan CM: Results of arthroscopic reduction and percutaneous fixation for acute displaced scaphoid fractures. *Arthroscopy* 2005;21:620-626.

CHAPTER 5

TREATMENT OF SCAPHOID NONUNIONS

ALEXANDER Y. SHIN, MD
ALLEN T. BISHOP, MD

The incidence of scaphoid nonunions has been reported to be between 5% and 15%,[1,2] with an estimate of 34,000 nonunions occurring per year in the United States.[3] The initial fracture, which typically occurs in an active adolescent or young adult, often is dismissed as a wrist sprain or never examined by a doctor. In the early stages, scaphoid nonunions are rarely symptomatic, and become symptomatic only when there is acute on chronic trauma, or when the wrist is stressed beyond normal activities.[2,4-6] Because treatment for scaphoid nonunions typically is surgical, it is important to understand that the successful surgical management is often related to early diagnosis and restoration of anatomy and carpal alignment, which can preserve carpal function and prevent the ultimate sequelae of degenerative wrist arthritis.

NATURAL HISTORY

The natural history of the undiagnosed or missed scaphoid fracture remains a controversial topic; it is impossible to accurately estimate how long a patient has had a nonunion because many patients are either asymptomatic or never seek treatment. In an attempt to determine the natural history of symptomatic scaphoid nonunions, Mack and colleagues[4] reviewed 46 military personnel with 47 scaphoid nonunions. Follow-up after the initial scaphoid fracture ranged from 5 to 53 years. The authors reported three distinct groups of patients with degenerative wrist arthritis.[4] Grade I wrists had changes confined to the scaphoid, typically cyst formation, fracture site resorption, and sclerosis that occurred

at an average of 8.2 years after fracture (**Figure 1,** *A* and *B*) . Grade II wrists demonstrated radiostyloid beaking with radiocarpal arthritis and occurred at an average of 17 years after fracture (**Figure 1,** *C* and *D*). Grade III wrists demonstrated progressive periscaphoid arthritis and occurred at an average of 31.6 years after fracture (**Figure 1,** *E* and *F*). Ruby and associates[5] confirmed Mack's findings in a study of 55 patients with 56 nonunions. Patients with fewer than 4 years of nonunion duration had a lower incidence of arthritis compared with those with more than 5 years' nonunion duration (9% versus 97% with arthritis). The authors concluded that the degree of arthritic changes was proportional to the duration of the nonunion and that the radiolunate, triquetrohamate articulations were spared. More recently, Martini[7] compared 41 patients with untreated nonunions with a group of 55 patients who underwent the Matti-Russe procedure (inlay bone graft). Surgical patients had better long-term results. Martini also noted that duration of nonunion and location were main determinants in the development of arthrosis and that no patient was free of arthrosis after 10 years of a nonunion. His recommendation based on this study was that nonunions should be treated as soon as possible to prevent secondary arthrosis.

The existence of asymptomatic scaphoid nonunions confounds the determination of the injury's natural history. Because only symptomatic nonunions presented to Mack and associates[4] and Ruby and associates,[5] the natural history is that of symptomatic nonunions and not all nonunions. The lack of a cohort of asymptomatic nonunions may have biased these studies, overstating

FIGURE 1

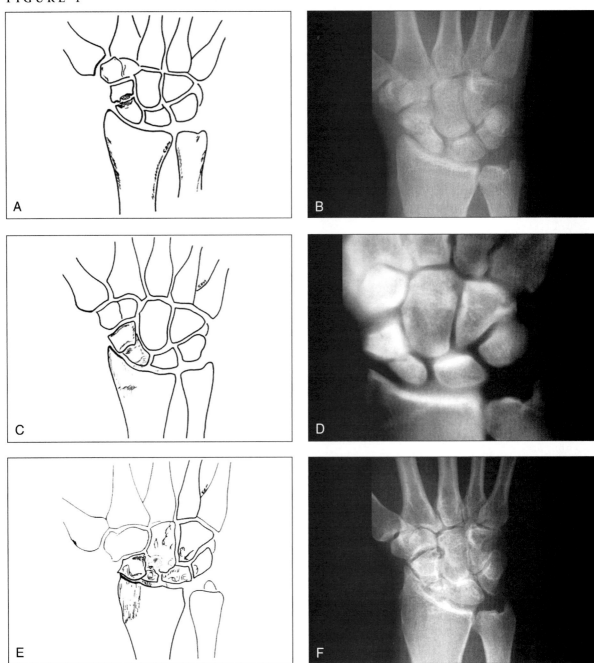

Mack classification of scaphoid nonunion advanced collapse. Diagram **(A)** and PA radiograph **(B)** show grade I wrists in which changes are confined to the scaphoid and typically consist of cyst formation, fracture site resorption, and sclerosis that occur at an average of 8.2 years after fracture. Diagram **(C)** and PA radiograph **(D)** show grade II wrists demonstrating radiostyloid beaking with radiocarpal arthritis that occur at an average of 17 years after fracture. Diagram **(E)** and PA radiograph **(F)** show grade III wrists demonstrating progressive periscaphoid arthritis that occur at an average of 31.6 years following fracture. (Figures **A, C,** and **E,** reproduced with permission from Mack GR, Bosse MJ, Gelberman RH, Yu E: The natural history of scaphoid nonunion. *J Bone Joint Surg Am* 1984;66:504-509.)

FIGURE 2

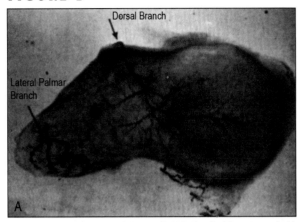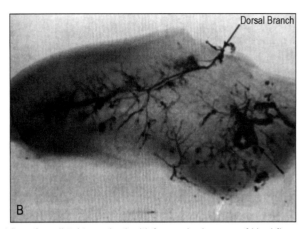

The intrinsic blood supply of the scaphoid is fragile. The retrograde blood flows from distal to proximal, with few proximal sources of blood flow, rendering the proximal fragment of the scaphoid fracture prone to avascular changes. The scaphoid intrinsic blood supply is via the lateral palmar branch **(A)** and dorsal branch **(B)**. (Reproduced with permission from Gelberman RH, Menon J: The vascularity of the scaphoid bone. *J Hand Surg Am* 1980;5:508-513.)

poor outcomes of untreated scaphoid nonunions.[7-10] Despite these reservations, a large number of patients with unstable scaphoid nonunions present with wrist pain, instability, and arthritic changes. For this reason, early and aggressive surgical treatment is recommended to prevent the late sequelae of instability and irreversible arthritic changes.

RISK FACTORS

The most frequently cited factor for the development of scaphoid nonunions is the tenuous retrograde blood supply[11-13] (**Figure 2**). In addition to the tenuous blood supply, 80% of the scaphoid is covered by cartilage. By definition, any fracture of the scaphoid is intra-articular, increasing the risk of both pseudarthrosis and arthritis. As the link between the distal and proximal carpal rows, the scaphoid acts as a slider crank stabilizer for the wrist and has tremendous forces placed against it. Fisk,[14] in his Huntarian Lectures, recognized scaphoid fracture leading to nonunion as a cause of carpal instability. The unfavorable biomechanics of the fractured scaphoid places this carpal bone at a significant risk for nonunion—the proximal scaphoid rotates dorsally into extension and the distal scaphoid flexes.[15] The lunate and proximal pole of the scaphoid extend into a dorsal intercalated segmental instability (DISI) pattern as described by Linscheid and colleagues[16] (**Figure 3**). Left untreated, the capitate pushes into the nonunion gap and further displaces the fracture fragments. Ultimately, degenerative changes occur as described.

Other risk factors for development of nonunion of acute fractures include delay of diagnosis and adequate treatment,[9] carpal collapse,[3] loss of scaphoid architecture,[17] or fracture displacement.[18]

DIAGNOSIS AND EVALUATION

The most common presentation of scaphoid nonunion is pain and loss of wrist motion. The pain is often a vague ache in the wrist that is exacerbated by loaded wrist extension and often necessitates modifications of the manner in which patients use their wrists (eg, use of a fist to open doors instead of a dorsiflexed wrist and flat palm). Most often, the time at which the fracture occurred is forgotten, and the injury often is dismissed as a wrist sprain that eventually becomes relatively asymptomatic until arthritic changes or a secondary injury occurs. Because of this, the duration of the scaphoid nonunion is often unknown.

Diagnosis of scaphoid nonunion is radiographic. Multiple view plain radiographs are initially obtained, and often a scaphoid nonunion is an incidental finding during radiographic examination of another part of the

FIGURE 3

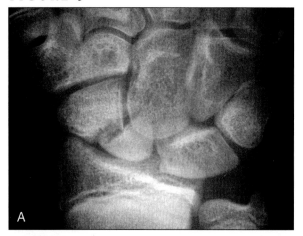

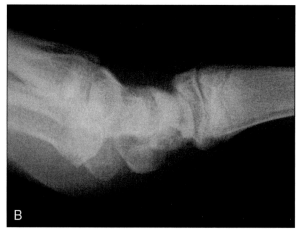

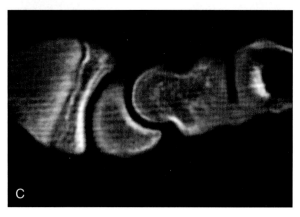

A break in the integrity of the proximal carpal row within the scaphoid can result in a DISI pattern similar to that of a scapholunate ligament disruption. This example of a scaphoid fracture resulting in the DISI deformity is shown in PA **(A)** and lateral **(B)** radiographs and a coronal CT scan **(C)**. (Courtesy of Mayo Clinic, 2006.)

hand. Radiology of scaphoid fractures and nonunions is described in a separate chapter. Briefly, multiple plain radiographs of the scaphoid should be obtained, including posteroanterior (PA), lateral, scaphoid (PA view with the wrist in 30° of extension and 20° of ulnar deviation, and oblique (in 45°of pronation) views (**Figure 4**). Careful radiographic evaluation of the lateral view will determine if a carpal collapse pattern exists (DISI). Additionally, the degree of arthritic changes, the vascular status of the proximal pole, and the degree of cyst formation or resorption of the nonunion site should be evaluated.

Often, plain radiographs are equivocal in diagnosing scaphoid nonunions and CT is needed to clearly define the fracture nonunion. In addition to defining the bony architecture, the CT scan is helpful in preoperative plan-

ning (**Figure 5**). Amadio and associates[17] described a method of quantifying carpal collapse by a measurement of intrascaphoid angles. The mean normal lateral interscaphoid angle is less than 30° and the mean anteroposterior interscaphoid angle is less than 40° (**Figure 6**). The authors reported that a lateral intrascaphoid angle of greater than 45° is associated with an increased incidence of arthrosis, even if the fracture is healed. An additional measure that can be obtained by CT is the height-to-length ratio measured on the sagittal scans.[19,20] Bain and colleagues[19] reported that a height-to-length ratio of more than 0.65 corresponds with significant carpal collapse. Finally, CT scans are invaluable in the assessment of postoperative healing.

The utility of MRI continues to evolve and improve with the various sequences and use of contrast; it has

FIGURE 4

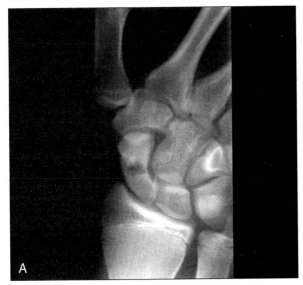
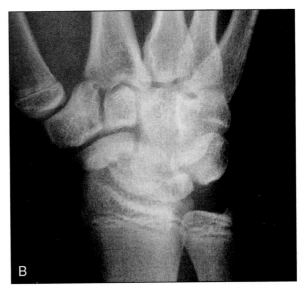

Scaphoid **(A)** and oblique **(B)** views in different patients render additional information regarding the scaphoid fracture and its geometry. (Courtesy of Mayo Clinic, 2006.)

FIGURE 5

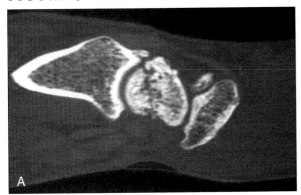
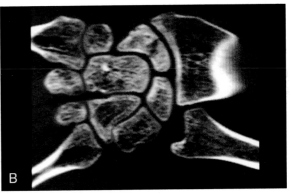

Sagittal **(A)** and coronal **(B)** CT reconstructions are invaluable in delineating the bony architecture and three-dimensional nuances of the scaphoid fracture nonunion. Sagittal reconstructions are particularly useful in identifying a scaphoid humpback deformity. (Courtesy of Mayo Clinic, 2006.)

been useful in the evaluation of proximal pole vascularity and should be included in the radiographic studies before surgical treatment (**Figure 7**). Cerezal and associates[21] compared gadolinium-enhanced MRI findings of the proximal pole of 30 patients with scaphoid nonunions with surgical findings and demonstrated 66% sensitivity, 88% specificity, and 83% accuracy. The correlation with surgical findings of osteonecrosis was statistically significant. Contrast-enhanced MRI demonstrates compromised vascularity[21] as well as early union and revascularization after surgery.[22]

MANAGEMENT OF SCAPHOID UNIONS

Once the diagnosis of a scaphoid nonunion is made, the decision to surgically treat the nonunion or to salvage the wrist needs to be made. It is important to recognize

FIGURE 6

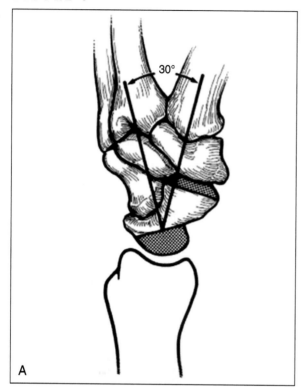
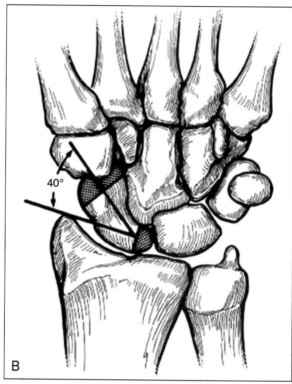

Intrascaphoid angles are useful in quantifying the degree of carpal collapse. The mean normal lateral interscaphoid angle **(A)** is less than 30° and the mean AP interscaphoid angle **(B)** is less than 40°. (Reproduced with permission from Amadio PC, Taleisnik J: Fractures of the carpal bones, in Green DP (ed): *Operative Hand Surgery*, ed. 3. New York, NY, Churchill Livingstone, 1993, pp 799-860.)

FIGURE 7

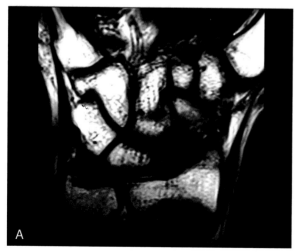
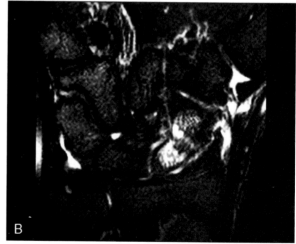

MRI scans demonstrate signal change consistent with avascular changes of the proximal pole of the scaphoid. **A,** T1-weighted image with decreased signal in the proximal scaphoid fragment, which is confirmed by a STIR image **(B)** demonstrating increased signal of the same fragment. (Courtesy of Mayo Clinic, 2006.)

that although there are reports of successfully uniting scaphoid nonunions with electrical stimulation and cast immobilization, with union rates reported as high as 69%,[23,24] most hand surgeons recommend open reduction and internal fixation of the nonunion combined with bone grafting.[2,4,7,10,25-45]

The decision to surgically fix a scaphoid nonunion hinges on several key factors, including the vascular status of the proximal pole, the presence or absence of degenerative arthritis, nonunion location, the degree of displacement of the fracture fragments, the presence or absence of carpal deformity, and patient-specific factors, such as age, occupation, and socioeconomic status.

Plain radiographs as well as CT scans should be carefully evaluated for arthritic changes at the radial styloid and midcarpal joint. Any evidence of arthritic change is a contraindication for surgical reconstruction, and salvage procedures should be considered. However, in the physiologically young patient with minimal radiostyloid changes, reconstruction with or without a radial styloidectomy should be considered; a salvage procedure always can be performed later.

In the absence of arthritic changes, or if the decision has been made to reconstruct the scaphoid with minimal articular changes, the next determinant of treatment is the vascular status of the proximal pole. Radiographs, CT, and gadolinium-enhanced MRI can give clues to the vascular status of the proximal pole, although none of these studies is foolproof, despite the favorable reports described. Intraoperative assessment of the proximal pole vascular status is imperative. Green[46] described punctuate bleeding from the proximal pole as evidence of proximal pole viability. Any suspected avascular changes in the proximal pole must be discussed with the patient, and alternative surgical plans should be made if the surgical findings do not corroborate findings on preoperative imaging.

The location of the nonunion determines the surgical approach. Proximal pole fractures are best approached dorsally; waist fractures are most effectively approached volarly. These are general guidelines, however, and it must be understood that each nonunion needs to be assessed individually to determine the optimal surgical approach. Occasionally, both a dorsal and volar approach may be required when there is significant deformity or abnormal bone growth.

The final determinants of treatment include the degree of fracture displacement and the degree of carpal deformity. The goals of surgical reconstruction are to restore the normal alignment and geometry of the scaphoid. A significant carpal collapse requires an interpositional bone graft to restore normal geometry. Similarly, significantly displaced fracture fragments need to be reduced as anatomically as possible.

Scaphoid nonunions that persist despite attempts at surgical intervention fall into a category of their own. These scaphoid nonunions can be particularly challenging because often there is loosening of the previously placed scaphoid screw with associated bone loss and carpal collapse. In these cases, the principles of evaluation of the degree of arthritis, vascularity of the proximal pole, and degree of collapse remain the same. When possible, revision scaphoid nonunion surgery should be attempted unless there is compelling evidence that the nonunion is unsalvageable. Smith and Cooney[40] reported on failed bone grafting of scaphoid nonunions treated with revision bone grafting in 25 patients treated at the Mayo Clinic. Of 19 scaphoids, 15 (79%) went on to union with revision bone grafting, which included 4 vascularized bone grafts and 11 conventional bone grafts (cancellous and wedge). Despite a 79% revision union rate, only 16% of patients were very satisfied and 8% moderately satisfied; there were only three excellent and five good results. Inoue and Kuwahata[47] reported on eight bone grafted scaphoid nonunions that failed and were treated with revision bone grafting and screw fixation. They united six of the eight nonunions. More recently, Preisser and associates[48] reported on 30 scaphoid nonunions in which previous surgery failed and thus required revision, and they demonstrated that only 64% were able to be united with revision surgery. A thorough discussion with these patients is mandatory so that they understand that although union of the scaphoid is possible, pain and functional limitations can persist.

SURGICAL RECONSTRUCTION
Bone Grafting

Although many different techniques have been described for treatment of scaphoid nonunions, the basic principles are the same, including meticulous débridement of necrotic nonviable and fibrous tissues, realignment of

FIGURE 8

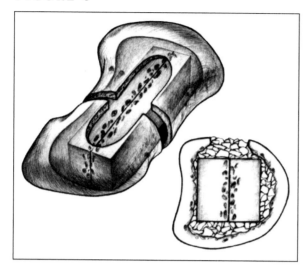

The volar approach to the scaphoid with bicortical bone graft for scaphoid nonunion was popularized by Russe. (Reproduced with permission from Green DP: Russe technique, in Gelberman RH (ed): *Master Techniques in Orthopaedic Surgery: The Wrist.* New York, NY, Raven Press, pp 107-118.)

FIGURE 9

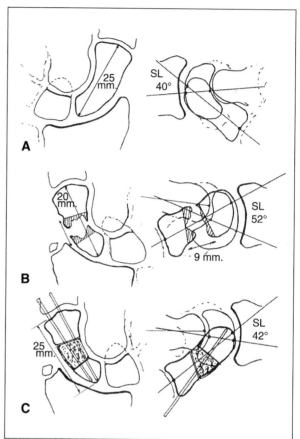

Volar interposition wedge graft to restore normal scaphoid geometry. **A,** Tracing of the uninjured wrist and measurement of scaphoid length and scapholunate (SL) angle. **B,** Calculation of the size of the resection area and form of graft. **C,** The operation. (Reproduced with permission from Fernandez DL: A technique for anterior wedge-shaped grafts for scaphoid nonunions with carpal instability. *J Hand Surg Am* 1984;9:733-737.)

the displaced fragments, and liberal use of bone graft (nonvascularized or vascularized) to fill the void, followed by rigid fixation whenever possible.

In 1936, Matti[49] described the dorsal inlay bone graft. Russe[50] described the volar approach to the scaphoid and use of a bicortical bone graft in 1960 (**Figure 8**). Both of these methods have been used in scaphoids without carpal collapse and only minimal displacement. In addressing carpal collapse associated with scaphoid nonunions, Fisk[14] recommended placement of a volar wedge graft to restore the normal scaphoid geometry, and the technique was subsequently perfected and reported by Fernandez[51] (**Figure 9**).

In 1984, Herbert and Fisher[52] reported the results of a headless compression screw that improved outcomes by affording rigid compression of the nonunion fragments. Soon after, a cannulated version was designed by Whipple and Herbert, with the result of accurate placement of the screw within the scaphoid. Subsequently, a plethora of headless cannulated screw designs have emerged. Whenever possible, screw fixation should be performed. There are, however, situations where Kirschner wire (K-wire) fixation is still needed secondary to the small fragment size.

Iliac Crest Wedge Graft With Arteriovenous Bundle Implantation

Hori and associates[53] demonstrated surgical angiogenesis of autogenous bone when an arteriovenous (AV) bundle was implanted into bone in a canine model. Since then, implantation of vessels has been shown to induce neovascularization and new bone formation not only in experimental animal models,[54-56] but also in the

FIGURE 10

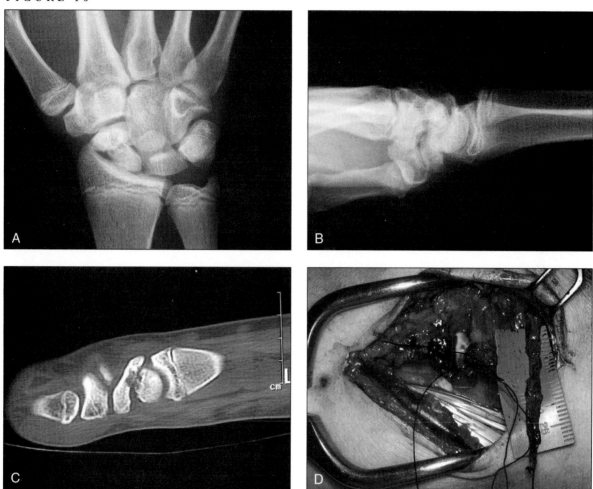

PA **(A)** and lateral **(B)** radiographs and a coronal CT scan **(C)** of a 14-year-old boy with open distal radius growth plates with a scaphoid nonunion with significant carpal collapse and humpback deformity. Intraoperatively, avascular compromise of the proximal scaphoid pole was found. An AV pedicle is harvested from the dorsal intercarpal arch **(D)**. (Courtesy of Mayo Clinic, 2006.)

human for Kienböck's disease,[57] talus osteonecrosis,[53] scaphoid nonunion with osteonecrosis,[58,59] and in prefabricated bone grafts.[60-63]

In 1995, Fernandez and Eggli[59] reported 11 patients with scaphoid nonunions treated with interposition iliac crest bone grafting with a second metacarpal artery AV pedicle implanted into the avascular proximal pole. Ten of the 11 nonunions were healed at an average of 10 weeks. One of the 10 united scaphoids failed secondary to radioscaphoid debilitating pain.

A variety of AV bundles can be used and include the second metacarpal artery/vein, the dorsal intercarpal arch (**Figure 10**), 4+5 extensor compartment artery, and so on.[64] Nearly any AV bundle with proper length can be used. Arteriovenous bundle implantation can be useful in restoring blood supply to a compromised proximal pole. If the scaphoid is collapsed (humpback deformity), an interposition wedge graft can be used to restore the normal scaphoid geometry, and an AV bundle can be placed into the proximal pole.

FIGURE 10 (CONT)

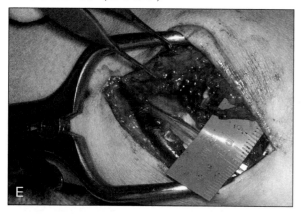

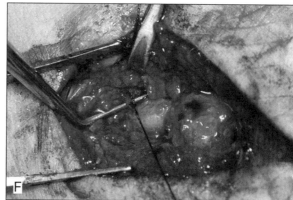

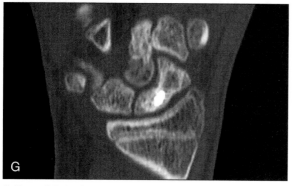

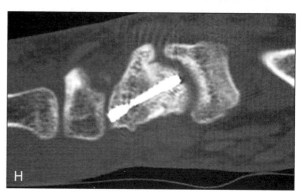

E, The pedicle is placed into the proximal scaphoid through a drill hole after an interposition wedge grafting and screw fixation is performed. **F,** The silk tie comes through the volar proximal scaphoid pole proximal to the iliac crest wedge graft. PA **(G)** and lateral **(H)** CT scans obtained 15 weeks after surgery demonstrate union and revascularization. (Courtesy of Mayo Clinic, 2006.)

Vascularized Bone Grafting

The concept of vascularized bone grafts for reconstruction of bone defects or osteonecrosis is nearly a century old. In 1905, Huntington[65] transferred a fibula with its nutrient artery pedicle for reconstruction of a tibial defect. It was not until 60 years later that Roy-Camille[66] transferred a pedicled vascularized bone graft (scaphoid tubercle) on an abductor pollicis brevis muscle pedicle to a delayed scaphoid fracture union. Vascularized bone grafts, unlike conventional bone grafts, preserve the circulation, as well as viable osteoclasts and osteoblasts. This allows primary bone healing without creeping substitution of dead bone.[67] Application of vascularized bone grafts to scaphoid nonunions with avascular proximal poles may aid or accelerate healing, replace deficient bone, and/or revascularize ischemic bone. The results reported to date have been promising.[66-77] (RM Braun, MD, San Diego, CA, unpublished paper presented at the American Society for Surgery of the Hand annual meeting, 1983.)

There are essentially two types of vascularized bone grafts used for the scaphoid: pedicled grafts and free vascularized grafts. The number of pedicled vascularized bone grafts for the scaphoid continues to grow (**Table 1**).[32,37-42,53,59,70,74,75,78-85] Our preference is the use of the 1,2 intercompartmental supraretinacular artery (ICRSA) vascularized bone graft. The anatomy of the dorsal distal radius has been extensively described as have the surgical techniques.[31,64,77] Free vascularized bone grafts used for the scaphoid include the iliac crest bone graft with associated deep circumflex iliac artery and venae comitantes[78,79] as well as the medial femoral condyle graft based on the descending genicular artery.[37]

FIGURE 11

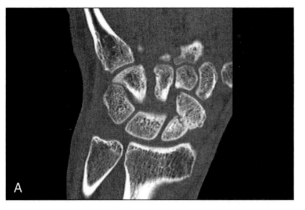

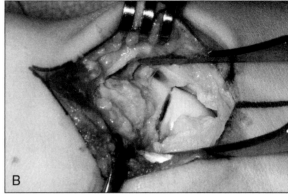

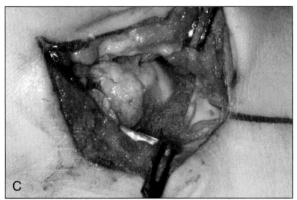

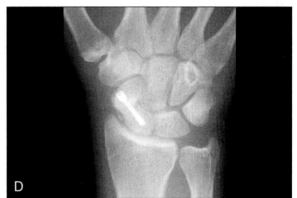

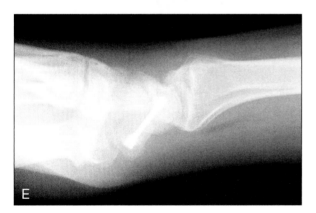

A coronal CT reconstruction **(A)** of a 15-year-old boy shows a scaphoid waist nonunion without osteonecrosis or carpal deformity. The nonunion was treated through a volar approach **(B)**, with curettage of the nonunion with iliac crest bone grafting **(C)**, and screw fixation. PA **(D)** and lateral **(E)** radiographs obtained 6 weeks postoperatively show healing of the nonunion. (Courtesy of Mayo Clinic, 2006.)

TREATMENT OPTIONS
No Osteonecrosis, No Carpal Deformity

In cases of scaphoid nonunion in which the proximal pole is viable and there is no carpal collapse or arthritic changes, cancellous bone grafting of the scaphoid nonunion with screw fixation is preferred (**Figure 11**). The surgical approach to the scaphoid depends on the location of the fracture nonunion. Waist nonunions are typically addressed via a volar Russe approach, whereas proximal pole nonunions require a dorsal approach.

TABLE 1

Results of Vascularized Bone Graft, With or Without Internal Fixation

Author(s) (Year)	Number of Nonunions	Graft Donor Site	Type of Internal Fixation	Length of Immobilization	Union		Comments and Complications
					%	95% CI	
Hori, et al (1979)	1	Cancellous bone		NA	100		Vascular bundle of dorsal index artery
Braun (1983)	5	Distal radius	K-wires	NA	80	(28-100)	Pronator quadratus pedicle blood supply
Kuhlmann, et al (1987)	3	Distal radius	K-wires	12	100	(29-100)	All had prior failed surgery for nonunion
Pechlaner, et al (1987	25	Ilium	K-wires	8	100	(86-100)	Most with necrotic proximal pole
Kawai and Yamamoto (1988)	8	Distal radius	K-wires	9	100	(63-100)	Pronator quadratus pedicle blood supply
Guimberteau and Panconi (1990)	8	Distal ulna		12	100	(63-100)	All thrid or fourth procedures
Zaidemberg, et al (1991)	11	Distal radius	K-wires	6	100	(72-100)	All long-standing nonunions
Fernandez and Eggli (1995)	11	Ilium	K-wires	10	91	(59-100)	Vascular bundle of dorsal index artery
Smith and Cooney (1996)	4	Distal radius	K-wires		100	(40-100)	All second procedures
Yuceturk, et al (1997)	4	First MC	Screw or K-wires	12	100	(40-100)	None with prior surgical attempts
Boyer, et al (1998)	10	Distal radius	Herbert screw	12	60	(26-88)	Additional K-wire; all necrosis of pole
Mathoulin and Brunelli (1998)	15	Second MC	K-wires	12	93	(68-100)	All second procedures
Mathoulin and Haerle (1998)	17	Distal radius	Herbert screw	9	100	(81-100)	Additional K-wire; 10 had prior surgery
Gabl, et al (1999)	15	Iliac crest	K-wires	12	80	(52-96)	All with an avascular proximal pole

TABLE 1(CONT)

Results of Vascularized Bone Graft, With or Without Internal Fixation

Author(s) (Year)	Number of Nonunions	Graft Donor Site	Type of Internal Fixation	Length of Immobilization	Union		Comments and Complications
					%	95% CI	
Gabl, et al (1999)	56	Iliac crest		12	85	(74-94)	Follow-up 8.8 years
Doi, et al (2000)	10	Distal femur	K-wires	6	100	(69-100)	All with an avascular proximal pole
Uerpairojkit, et al (2000)	10	Distal radius	Screws or K-wires	6	100	(69-100)	Five with an avascular proximal pole
Harpf, et al (2001)	60	Iliac crest	K-wires	12	92	(82-97)	Twenty-six with an avascular proximal pole
Malizos, et al (2001)	22	Distal radius	K-wires	8	100	(85-100)	All long-standing nonunions
Steinmann, et al (2002)	14	Distal radius	Screw or K-wires	11	100	(77-100)	Five second procedures; Eight proximal
Straw, et al (2002)	22	Distal radius	Screw or K-wires	7-12	27	(11-50)	Vascularization of the bone graft may not improve the union rate
Totals	331			10	91	(87-94)	

(Reproduced with permission from Munk B, Larsen CF: Bone grafting the scaphoid nonunion: A systematic review of 147 publications including 5,246 cases of scaphoid nonunion. *Acta Orthop Scand* 2004; 75: 618-629.)

Because there is no deformity, cancellous bone graft can be placed into the nonunion site after creating a trough in the volar scaphoid waist and curetting the nonunion site of fibrous debris. Rigid fixation with a headless cannulated screw is preferred. Proximal pole nonunions with vascular proximal poles without carpal collapse are relatively uncommon, but do occur. In these cases, disturbing the nonunion site may lead to avascular changes in the proximal fragment and as such, screw fixation without bone grafting may be preferred. Finally, arthroscopic screw placement and bone grafting through an arthroscope placed into the drilled hole of the scaphoid has been described by Slade and Dodds.[86]

No Osteonecrosis, Carpal Deformity

When carpal deformity is present without osteonecrosis of the proximal pole, restoration of the normal geometry of the scaphoid is recommended. The typical deformity associated with scaphoid waist nonunions is extension of the proximal pole and remainder of the proximal carpal row with flexion of the distal scaphoid fragment. The resultant DISI collapse shortens the carpus and alters the biomechanics of the wrist. Restoration of the length and flexion deformity of the scaphoid is recommended (**Figure 12**). As described by Fisk[14] and then popularized by Fernandez,[51] an interposition wedge

FIGURE 12

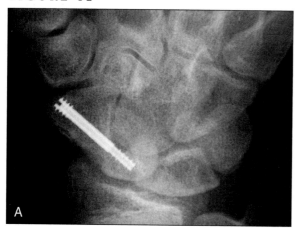
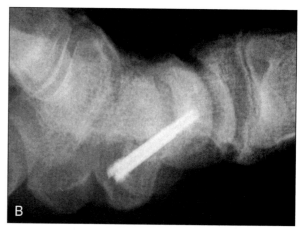

When there is no osteonecrosis but significant carpal collapse, as in the patient shown in Figure 3, restoration of normal scaphoid geometry is recommended. PA **(A)** and lateral **(B)** radiographs of the same patient obtained 12 weeks following iliac crest wedge grafting and screw fixation show union and restoration of normal carpal alignment. (Courttesy of Mayo Clinic, 2006.)

graft is placed to restore the normal scaphoid geometry followed by headless compression screw fixation.

Osteonecrosis, No Carpal Deformity, Proximal Nonunion

Proximal pole osteonecrosis without carpal deformity can be challenging to manage. There are several recommendations for this type of fracture nonunion, and most authors recommend some type of revascularization procedure. Based on our experience with vascularized bone grafts from the dorsal distal radius, we prefer the use of the 1,2 ICSRA vascularized bone graft (**Figure 13**).[43] Headless screw fixation improves union rates over K-wire fixation and should be used whenever possible. Other vascularized bone graft alternatives include the volar distal radius bone graft described by Mathoulin and Haerle[80] or the many other sources described in the literature.

Osteonecrosis, No Carpal Deformity, Waist

Treatment recommendations are not straightforward in patients with a scaphoid waist nonunion with avascular proximal pole and no carpal collapse. The recommendations in the literature vary and often can be confusing. Reports of vascularized bone grafts are highly encouraging; however, no prospective randomized series

have compared waist nonunions treated with traditional bone grafting versus vascularized bone grafting.[28,29] Our preference has been to perform vascularized bone grafting for these types of nonunions; however, the results of traditional bone grafting are compelling as well.

Osteonecrosis, Carpal Deformity

The most difficult situation is the combination of nonunion, proximal pole osteonecrosis, and carpal deformity. It is in these cases that structural graft and a vascular source are preferred over structural graft alone (**Figure 14**). There are essentially two methods that can deliver both structural graft and blood supply: (1) interposition iliac crest graft with implantation of an AV bundle into the proximal pole[59] and (2) free vascularized bone grafting with either iliac crest[78,79] or medial femoral condyle.[37] The results, indications, and outcomes for these procedures are detailed in the next section. Suffice it to say that the complexity of the scaphoid reconstruction is maximized and requires surgeons with microsurgical expertise to harvest and anastomose the vessels.

Previously Failed Nonunion Surgery

Previously failed nonunion surgery can be challenging and requires careful evaluation of radiographs and CT scans, as well as discussion of salvage procedures. With

FIGURE 13

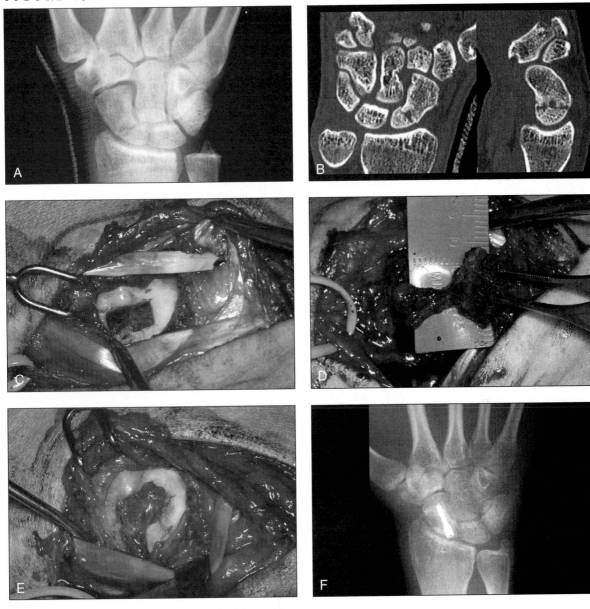

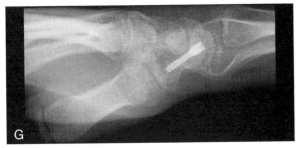

PA radiograph **(A)** and coronal CT scan **(B)** of a 31-year-old man who has a proximal pole scaphoid nonunion with osteonecrosis and no evidence of carpal collapse. The scaphoid nonunion is prepared with a trough across the nonunion site **(C)**, after which the 1,2 ICSRA bone graft is harvested **(D)**, and inset into the nonunion site **(E)**. Screw fixation is performed when possible. PA **(F)** and lateral **(G)** radiographs obtained 12 weeks postoperatively show union. (Courtesy of Mayo Clinic, 2006.)

FIGURE 14

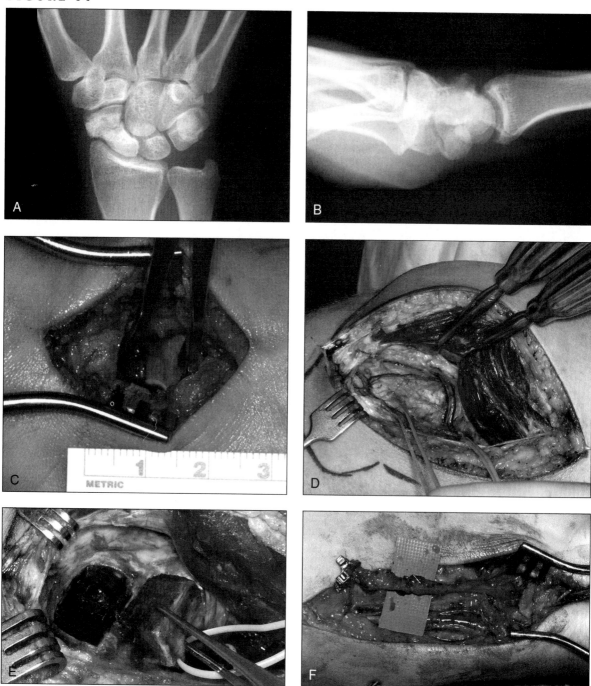

PA **(A)** and lateral **(B)** radiographs of a 22-year-old man who presents with osteonecrosis and a significant humpback deformity following previously failed surgery. A volar approach is used, and an intraoperative photograph **(C)** shows the humpback deformity. **D,** A medial femoral condyle vascularized bone graft based on the descending genicular artery. **E,** A large structurally sound piece of corticocancellous bone with excellent blood supply is harvested. **F,** The bone graft is inset and screw fixation is performed. (Courtesy of Mayo Clinic, 2006.)

FIGURE 14 (CONT)

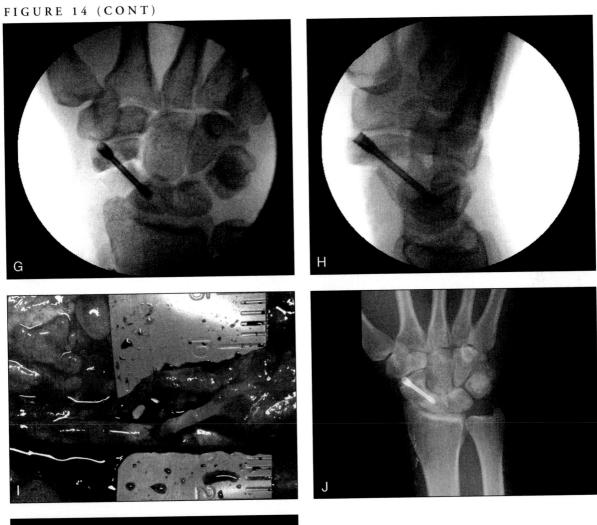

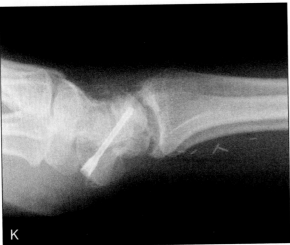

Intraoperative fluoroscopic PA **(G)** and lateral **(H)** images confirm screw placement, after which time vascular anastomosis to the radial artery and venae commitantes is performed **(I)**. PA **(J)** and lateral **(K)** radiographs obtained 15 weeks postoperatively show union. (Courtesy of Mayo Clinic, 2006.)

reported union rates ranging between 64% and 79% of revision of failed nonunion surgery,[40] we recommend attempts at revision surgery when possible. The articular cartilage must be carefully evaluated and if damaged, salvage procedures should be pursued. Technical challenges exist when the previously placed screw has cut out or has created significant defects. If avascular changes and carpal collapse exist, use of free vascularized bone grafts may be required to restore carpal alignment and vascularity to the proximal poles. The options of salvage procedures also should be carefully discussed.

OUTCOMES

Despite the numerous reports in the literature regarding the results of treatment of scaphoid nonunions, distilling the results to apply to a specific nonunion type (eg, location, with or without osteonecrosis, with or without carpal collapse, previous surgery) is difficult. Prospective randomized controlled studies of similar scaphoid nonunions with a defined postoperative protocol are lacking. Based on a review and meta-analyses of the literature, the following represent the results of treatment by graft typed used.

Conventional Grafting

The first description of a surgical treatment of a scaphoid nonunion bone grafting was by Adams and Leonard[87] in 1928; they successfully united a scaphoid nonunion with tibial bone graft. Controversy in the utility of this procedure was evident when in 1935, Cole and Williamson[88] stated that "bone grafting of the fragments has been done with some success but will never be a choice for routine procedure and it is mainly a surgical stunt." Over the next two decades, attitudes toward surgical treatment of scaphoid nonunions changed, mostly secondary to the contributions of Matti[49] and Russe.[50]

Conventional bone grafting is defined by use of bone graft that is nonvascularized and can be used as an inlay graft as described by Russe[50] and Matti[49] or an interposition wedge graft to restore scaphoid length and fix humpback deformity. Additionally, treatment can be with or without internal fixation. The results of treatment vary with nonunion type as well as whether or not internal fixation is used.

In a meta-analysis of the literature, Merrell and associates[28] demonstrated that of the 1,121 published articles by 2002, only 36 articles met the inclusion criteria to allow a quantitative analysis. From these 36 articles, which included 1,827 scaphoid nonunion repairs, the authors concluded the following regarding conventional bone grafting of unstable nonunions (with carpal collapse or displacement): Screw fixation with grafting resulted in better results (94% union) versus K-wires and wedge grafting (77% union; P < 0.01). However, in the presence of proximal avascular changes, these authors demonstrated that the union rate with conventional wedge grafting and screw fixation dropped to 47%.

Another meta-analysis by Munk and Larsen[29] demonstrated that nonvascularized bone graft without internal fixation yielded a union rate of 80% with a 95% confidence interval of 77% to 82%. These authors also noted that nonvascularized bone graft with internal fixation (K-wires, staples, or screw) yielded a union rate of 84% with a 95% confidence interval of 82% to 85%.

Vascularized Bone Grafting

In the event that the proximal pole is avascular, the use of vascularized bone grafts to restore vascularity to the proximal pole is intuitive. In 1965, Judet[89] made the simple observation that "dead bone added to dead bone does not produce living bone." Overall union rates of vascularized bone grafting for scaphoid nonunions has been reported to be 91% by one meta-analysis.[29] It is important to understand that the union rate differs on the status of the vascularity of the proximal pole and the location of the nonunion (proximal pole or waist). Merrell and associates[28] reported that in the presence of osteonecrosis, vascularized bone grafts resulted in an 88% union rate.

1,2-Intercompartmental Supraretinacular Artery

The use of the 1,2 ICSRA was initially popularized by Zaidemberg and colleagues,[42] who reported the use of a dorsal radial pedicle graft, achieving healing in 100% of 11 long-standing scaphoid nonunions. The vascular anatomy of the dorsal distal radius was defined by Sheetz and associates,[64] including an accurate description of Zaidemberg's graft among others from the dorsal distal radius of potential use in the carpus. The vessel originally described by Zaidemberg as the "ascending irrigating artery" is correctly described and named the 1,2-ICSRA. Union rates of 100% using the 1,2-ICSRA pedicled vascularized bone graft have been reported by several authors.[81-83,90] However, others have reported less-than-ideal healing rates using the same dorsal distal radius pedicled bone graft.[32,39]

In a critical analysis of the result of the 1,2 ICSRA vascularized bone graft, the Mayo Clinic group[43] reported on 48 patients with 49 scaphoid nonunions treated with this vascularized bone graft. In this very detailed report, the authors demonstrated a 71% overall union rate, with union occurring at an average of 15.6 weeks. Breaking down the various types of nonunions, the authors demonstrated a 50% union rate in proximal pole osteonecrosis compared with a 91% union if no osteonecrosis was present. Factors associated with failure included proximal pole avascularity, history of smoking tobacco (46% union rate in smokers versus 80% union in nonsmokers), type of fixation (screw fixation with a 88% union rate versus 53% union rate with K-wires), and carpal collapse (50% of failures had carpal collapse with a humpback deformity versus 11% of the failures occurred when there was no carpal collapse). The authors demonstrated that successful outcome is not universal with the 1,2 ICSRA graft and that careful selection of both patient and fracture is imperative.

Medial Femoral Condyle

The use of the medial femoral condyle as a source of vascularized bone graft was introduced by Hertel and Masquelet[91] in 1989. This vascularized bone graft allowed for a thin and flexible corticoperiosteal flap with a long vascular pedicle that allowed for broad coverage of bone defects, especially of long bones. In 2000, Doi and colleagues[37] reported on its use for scaphoid nonunions. These authors treated 10 patients with scaphoid nonunions associated with proximal pole osteonecrosis with the medial femoral condyle vascularized bone graft and obtained union in all patients at an average of 12 weeks postoperatively. The bone graft was an interposition wedge in all cases. Two of the 10 patients had subsequent radiocarpal arthritis and were dissatisfied with the outcome. Three of the patients had scapholunate angles greater than 62°, indicating a DISI deformity with carpal collapse. Donor site morbidity was minimal.

Unfortunately, there are no other reports of the use

of this type of vascularized bone graft for scaphoid nonunions to date.

Free Iliac Crest Bone Graft

Application of a free vascularized iliac crest bone graft to scaphoid nonunions was reported by the Insbruch group in 1999 and 2001.[78,79] In their 1999 report, the authors treated 15 patients with nonunions with proximal pole osteonecrosis with vascularized iliac crest bone graft and obtained union in 12 of 15. The technique used was an inlay graft via a volar approach. Scaphoids with collapse were not addressed in this series. In their 2001 report, 60 patients (21 with more than 4-year recalcitrance, 26 with proximal pole osteonecrosis, and 13 with previous surgery) were treated with this technique. The authors demonstrated an overall union rate of 91.7%. In the group with a more than 4-year duration of nonunion, 92% united. Union rate with proximal pole osteonecrosis was 90%; however, it should be noted that none of these patients had carpal collapse or humpback deformities. The previous surgery group had a union rate of 92%. Donor site morbidity was high, with a 55% incidence of hyperostosis of the iliac crest, 31.7% incidence of nerve hypesthesia, and 8.3% incidence of deformity of the iliac crest.

CONCLUSION

Treatment of scaphoid nonunions can be both rewarding and challenging. Early diagnosis and treatment, when possible, can avoid the late complications of the untreated scaphoid nonunion. When faced with treatment of a scaphoid nonunion, all factors must be evaluated, including fracture characteristics and patient factors. Although many options exist for the treatment of scaphoid nonunion, it is imperative to understand the outcomes, technical challenges, indications, and contraindications for each technique.

REFERENCES

1. Gellman H, Caputo RJ, Carter V, Aboulafia A, McKay M: Comparison of short and long thumb-spica casts for non-displaced fractures of the carpal scaphoid [see comments]. *J Bone Joint Surg Am* 1989;71:354-357.

2. Kuschner SH, Lane CS, Brien WW, Gellman H: Scaphoid fractures and scaphoid nonunion. Diagnosis and treatment. *Orthop Rev* 1994;23:861-871.

3. Osterman AL, Mikulics M: Scaphoid nonunion. *Hand Clin* 1988;4:437-455.

4. Mack GR, Bosse MJ, Gelberman RH, Yu E: The natural history of scaphoid nonunion. *J Bone Joint Surg Am* 1984;66:504-509.

5. Ruby LK, Stinson J, Belsky MR: The natural history of scaphoid nonunion. *J Bone Joint Surg Am* 1985;67:428-432.

6. Gelberman RH, Wolock BS, Siegel DB: Fractures and nonunions of the carpal scaphoid. *J Bone Joint Surg Am* 1989;71:1560-1565.

7. Martini AK: [Natural course in pseudarthrosis of the scaphoid]. *Orthopade* 1994;23:249-254.

8. Herbert TJ: Natural history of scaphoid nonunion: a critical analysis. *J Hand Surg Am* 1994;19:155-156.

9. Simonian PT, Trumble TE: Scaphoid nonunion. *J Am Acad Orthop Surg* 1994;2:185-191.

10. Kerluke L, McCabe SJ: Nonunion of the scaphoid: A critical analysis of recent natural history studies. *J Hand Surg Am* 1993;18:1-3.

11. Gelberman RH, Panagis JS, Taleisnik J, Baumgaertner M: The arterial anatomy of the human carpus. Part I: The extraosseous vascularity. *J Hand Surg* 1983;8:367-375.

12. Panagis JS, Gelberman RH, Taleisnik J, Baumgaertner M: The arterial anatomy of the human carpus. Part II: The intraosseous vascularity. *J Hand Surg* 1983;8:375-382.

13. Taleisnik J, Kelley PJ: The extraosseous and intraosseous blood supply of the scaphoid bone. *J Bone Joint Surg Am* 1966;48:1125-1137.

14. Fisk GR: Carpal instability and the fractured scaphoid. *Ann R Coll Surg Engl* 1970;46:63-76.

15. Smith DK, Cooney WP, An KN, Linscheid RL, Chao EYS: Effects of simulated unstable scaphoid fractures on carpal motion. *J Hand Surg Am* 1989;14:283-291.

16. Linscheid RL, Dobyns JH, Beabout JW, Bryan RS: Traumatic instability of the wrist: diagnosis, classification, and pathomechanics. *J Bone Joint Surg Am* 1972;54:1612.

17. Amadio PC, Berquist TH, Smith DK, Ilstrup DM, Cooney WP III, Linscheid RL: Scaphoid malunion. *J Hand Surg Am* 1989;14:679-687.

18. Eddeland A, Eiken O, Hellgren E, Ohlsson NM: Fractures of the scaphoid. *Scand J Plast Reconstr Surg* 1975;9:234-239.

19. Bain GI, Bennett JD, MacDermid JC, Slethaug GP, Richards RS, Roth JH: Measurement of the scaphoid humpback deformity using longitudinal computed tomography: Intra- and interobserver variability using various measurement techniques. *J Hand Surg Am* 1998;23:76-81.

20. Bain GI, Bennett JD, Richards RS, Slethaug GP, Roth JH: Longitudinal computed tomography of the scaphoid: A new technique. *Skeletal Radiol* 1995;24:271-273.

21. Cerezal L, Abascal F, Canga A, Garcia-Valtuille R, Bustamante M, del Pinal F: Usefulness of gadolinium-enhanced MR imaging in the evaluation of the vascularity of scaphoid nonunions. *AJR Am J Roentgenol* 2000;174:141-149.

22. Dailiana ZH, Zachos V, Varitimidis S, Papanagiotou P, Karantanas A, Malizos KN: Scaphoid nonunions treated with vascularised bone grafts: MRI assessment. *Eur J Radiol* 2004;50:217-224.

23. Adams BD, Frykman GK, Taleisnik J: Treatment of scaphoid nonunion with casting and pulsed electromagnetic fields: A study continuation. *J Hand Surg Am* 1992;17:910-914.

24. Frykman GK, Taleisnik J, Peters G, et al: Treatment of nonunited scaphoid fractures by pulsed electromagnetic field and cast. *J Hand Surg Am* 1986;11:344-349.

25. Daecke W, Wieloch P, Vergetis P, Jung M, Martini AK: Occurrence of carpal osteoarthritis after treatment of scaphoid nonunion with bone graft and Herbert screw: A long-term follow-up study. *J Hand Surg Am* 2005;30:923-931.

26. Dailiana ZH, Malizos KN, Zachos V, Varitimidis SE, Hantes M, Karantanas A: Vascularized bone grafts from the palmar radius for the treatment of waist nonunions of the scaphoid. *J Hand Surg Am* 2006;31:397-404.

27. Garcia-Mata S: Carpal scaphoid fracture nonunion in children. *J Pediatr Orthop* 2002;22:448-451.

28. Merrell GA, Wolfe SW, Slade JF III: Treatment of scaphoid nonunions: Quantitative meta-analysis of the literature. *J Hand Surg Am* 2002;27:685-691.

29. Munk B, Larsen CF: Bone grafting the scaphoid nonunion: A systematic review of 147 publications including 5,246 cases of scaphoid nonunion. *Acta Orthop Scand* 2004;75:618-629.

30. Pao VS, Chang J: Scaphoid nonunion: Diagnosis and treatment. *Plast Reconstr Surg* 2003;112:1666-1676; quiz 1677; discussion 1678-1669.

31. Shin AY, Bishop AT: Pedicled vascularized bone grafts for disorders of the carpus: Scaphoid nonunion and Kienbock's disease. *J Am Acad Orthop Surg* 2002;10:210-216.

32. Straw RG, Davis TR, Dias JJ: Scaphoid nonunion: Treatment with a pedicled vascularized bone graft based on the 1,2 intercompartmental supraretinacular branch of the radial artery. *J Hand Surg Br* 2002;27:413.

33. Trumble TE, Salas P, Barthel T, Robert KQ III: Management of scaphoid nonunions. *J Am Acad Orthop Surg* 2003;11:380-391.

34. Waters PM, Stewart SL: Surgical treatment of nonunion and avascular necrosis of the proximal part of the scaphoid in adolescents. *J Bone Joint Surg Am* 2002;84:915-920.

35. Trumble T, Nyland W: Scaphoid nonunions: Pitfalls and pearls. *Hand Clin* 2001;17:611-624.

36. Nagle DJ: Scaphoid nonunion: Treatment with cancellous bone graft and Kirschner-wire fixation. *Hand Clin* 2001;17:625-629.

37. Doi K, Oda T, Soo-Heong T, Nanda V: Free vascularized bone graft for nonunion of the scaphoid. *J Hand Surg Am* 2000;25:507-519.

38. Gabl M, Reinhart C, Pechlaner S, Hussl H: [Proximal scaphoid pseudarthrosis with avascular pole fragment: Long-term outcome after reconstruction with microvascular pedicled iliac crest bone graft]. *Handchir Mikrochir Plast Chir* 1999;31:196-199.

39. Boyer MI, von Schroeder HP, Axelrod TS: Scaphoid nonunion with avascular necrosis of the proximal pole: Treatment with a vascularized bone graft from the dorsum of the distal radius. *J Hand Surg Br* 1998;23:686-690.

40. Smith BS, Cooney WP: Revision of failed bone grafting for nonunion of the scaphoid: Treatment options and results. *Clin Orthop Relat Res* 1996:98-109.

41. Yuceturk A, Isiklar ZU, Tuncay C, Tandogan R: Treatment of scaphoid nonunions with a vascularized bone graft based on the first dorsal metacarpal artery. *J Hand Surg Br* 1997;22:425-427.

42. Zaidemberg C, Siebert JW, Angrigiani C: A new vascularized bone graft for scaphoid nonunion. *J Hand Surg Am* 1991;16:474-478.

43. Chang MA, Bishop AT, Moran SL, Shin AY: The outcomes and complications of 1,2-intercompartmental supraretinacular artery pedicled vascularized bone grafting of scaphoid nonunions. *J Hand Surg Am* 2006;31:387-396.

44. Cooney WP, Dobyns JH, Linscheid RL: Fractures of the scaphoid: A rational approach to management. *Clin Orthop* 1980:90-97.

45. Jupiter JB, Shin AY, Trumble TE, Fernandez DL: Traumatic and reconstructive problems of the scaphoid. *Instr Course Lect* 2001;50:105-122.

46. Green DP: The effect of avascular necrosis on Russe bone grafting for scaphoid nonunion. *J Hand Surg Am* 1985;10:579-605.

47. Inoue G, Kuwahata Y: Repeat screw stabilization with bone grafting after a failed Herbert screw fixation for acute scaphoid fractures and nonunions. *J Hand Surg Am* 1997;22:413-418.

48. Preisser P, Rudolf KD, Partecke BD: [Persistent scaphoid pseudarthrosis after surgical treatment: results of repeated bone transplantation]. *Handchir Mikrochir Plast Chir* 1999;31:187-195.

49. Matti H: Uber die Behandlung der Naviculare-Fraktur durch Plombierung mit Spongiosa. *Zbl Chir* 1937;64:2353-2359.

50. Russe O: Fracture of the carpal navicular: Diagnosis, nonoperative treatment, and operative treatment. *J Bone Joint Surg Am* 1960;42:759-768.

51. Fernandez DL: A technique for anterior wedge-shaped grafts for scaphoid nonunions with carpal instability. *J Hand Surg Am* 1984;9:733-737.

52. Herbert TJ, Fisher WE: Management of the fractured scaphoid using a new bone screw. *J Bone Joint Surg Br* 1984;66:114-123.

53. Hori Y, Tamai S, Okuda H, Sakamoto H, Takita T, Masuhara K: Blood vessel transplantation to bone. *J Hand Surg* 1979;4:23-33.

54. Sunagawa T, Bishop AT, Muramatsu K: Role of conventional and vascularized bone grafts in scaphoid nonunion with avascular necrosis: A canine experimental study. *J Hand Surg Am* 2000;25:849-859.

55. Suzuki O, Bishop AT, Sunagawa T, Katsube K, Friedrich PF: VEGF-promoted surgical angiogenesis in necrotic bone. *Microsurgery* 2004;24:85-91.

56. Busa R, Adani R, Castagnetti C, Zaffe D, Mingione A: Neovascularized bone grafts: Experimental investigation. *Microsurgery* 1999;19:289-295.

57. Tamai S, Yajima H, Ono H: Revascularization procedures in the treatment of Kienbock's disease. *Hand Clin* 1993;9:455-466.

58. Steinmann SP, Bishop AT: A vascularized bone graft for repair of scaphoid nonunion. *Hand Clin* 2001;17:647-653, ix.

59. Fernandez DL, Eggli S: Nonunion of the scaphoid: Revascularization of the proximal pole with implantation of a vascular bundle and bone grafting. *J Bone Joint Surg Am* 1995;77:883-893.

60. Khouri RK, Upton J, Shaw WW: Prefabrication of composite free flaps through staged microvascular transfer: An experimental and clinical study. *Plast Reconstr Surg* 1991;87:108-115.

61. Khouri RK, Koudsi B, Reddi H: Tissue transformation into bone in vivo : A potential practical application. *JAMA* 1991;266:1953-1955.

62. Hirase Y, Valauri FA, Buncke HJ: Neovascularized bone, muscle, and myo-osseous free flaps: An experimental model. *J Reconstr Microsurg* 1988;4:209-215.

63. Vinzenz KG, Holle J, Wuringer E, Kulenkampff KJ: Prefabrication of combined scapula flaps for microsurgical reconstruction in oro-maxillofacial defects: A new method. *J Craniomaxillofac Surg* 1996;24:214-223.

64. Sheetz KK, Bishop AT, Berger RA: The arterial blood supply of the distal radius and its potential use in vascularized pedicled bone grafts. *J Hand Surg Am* 1995;20:902-914.

65. Huntington TW: Case of bone transference. *Ann Surg* 1905;41:249-256.

66. Roy-Camille R: Fractures et pseudarthroses du scaphoide moyen: Utilisation d'un greffo pedicule. *Actual Chir Ortho R Poincare* 1965;4:197-214.

67. Barth H: Histologische untersuchungen uber knockentransplantation. *Beitr Pathol Anat Allg Pathol* 1895;17:65-142.

68. Fernandez DL: Anterior bone grafting and conventional lag screw fixation to treat scaphoid nonunions. *J Hand Surg Am* 1990;15:140-147.

69. Leung PC, Hung LK: Use of pronator quadratus bone flap in bony reconstruction around the wrist. *J Hand Surg Am* 1990;15:637-640.

70. Kawai H, Yamamoto K: Pronator quadratus pedicled bone graft for old scaphoid fractures. *J Bone Joint Surg Br* 1988;70:829-831.

71. Chacha PB: Vascularized pedicular bone grafts. *Int Orthop* 1984;8:117-138.

72. Beck E: Die verpflanzung des os pisiforme am gafassstiel zur behandlung der lunatummalazie. *Handchirurgie* 1971;3:64-67.

73. Beck E: Der os pisiforme-transfer. *Orthopade* 1986;15:131-134.

74. Guimberteau JC, Panconi B: Recalcitrant non-union of the scaphoid treated with a vascularized bone graft based on the ulnar artery. *J Bone Joint Surg Am* 1990;72:88-97.

75. Kuhlmann JN, Mimoun M, Boabighi A, Baux S: Vascularized bone graft pedicled on the volar carpal artery for non-union of the scaphoid. *J Hand Surg Br* 1987;12:203-210.

76. Saffar P: Remplacement du semi-lunaire par le pisiforme: Description d'une nouvelle technique pour le traitement de la maladie de kienbock. *Ann Chir Main* 1982;1:276-279.

77. Shin AY, Bishop AT, Berger RA: Vascularized pedicled bone grafts for disorders of the carpus. *Tech Hand Up Extrem Surg* 1998;2:94-109.

78. Gabl M, Reinhart C, Lutz M, et al: Vascularized bone graft from the iliac crest for the treatment of nonunion of the proximal part of the scaphoid with an avascular fragment. *J Bone Joint Surg Am* 1999;81:1414-1428.

79. Harpf C, Gabl M, Reinhart C, et al: Small free vascularized iliac crest bone grafts in reconstruction of the scaphoid bone: A retrospective study in 60 cases. *Plast Reconstr Surg* 2001;108:664-674.

80. Mathoulin C, Haerle M: Vascularized bone graft from the palmar carpal artery for treatment of scaphoid nonunion. *J Hand Surg Br* 1998;23:318-323.

81. Uerpairojkit C, Leechavengvongs S, Witoonchart K: Primary vascularized distal radius bone graft for nonunion of the scaphoid. *J Hand Surg Br* 2000;25:266-270.

82. Steinmann SP, Bishop AT, Berger RA: Use of the 1,2 intercompartmental supraretinacular artery as a vascularized pedicle bone graft for difficult scaphoid nonunion. *J Hand Surg Am* 2002;27:391-401.

83. Malizos KN, Dailiana ZH, Kirou M, Vragalas V, Xenakis TA, Soucacos PN: Longstanding nonunions of scaphoid fractures with bone loss: Successful reconstruction with vascularized bone grafts. *J Hand Surg Br* 2001;26:330-334.

84. Pechlaner S, Lohmann H, Buck-Gramcko D, Martin L: Pseudarthrosis of the scaphoid bone: Experiences in

240 cases. *Handchir Mikrochir Plast Chir* 1987;19:306-309.

85. Mathoulin C, Brunelli, F: Further experience with the index metacarpal vascularized bone graft. *J Hand Surg Br* 1998;23:311-317.

86. Slade JF III, Dodds SD: Minimally invasive management of scaphoid nonunions. *Clin Orthop Relat Res* 2006;445:108-119.

87. Adams JD, Leonard RD: Fracture of the carpal scaphoid: New method of treatment with report of one case. *N Engl J Med* 1928;198:401-404.

88. Cole WH, Williamson GA: Fractures of the carpal navicular bone. *Minn Med* 1935;18:81-83.

89. Judet RR-CR: Fractures et pseudoartrhoses du scaphoide moyen: Utilisation d'un greffon pedicule. *Actualites Chir Orthop* 1965;4.

90. Tsai TT, Chao EK, Tu YK, Chen AC, Lee MS, Ueng SW: Management of scaphoid nonunion with avascular necrosis using 1, 2 intercompartmental supraretinacular arterial bone grafts. *Chang Gung Med J* 2002;25:321-328.

91. Hertel R, Masquelet AC: The reverse flow medial knee osteoperiosteal flap for skeletal reconstruction of the leg: Description and anatomical basis. *Surg Radiol Anat* 1989;11:257-262.

CHAPTER 6

TRANSSCAPHOID PERILUNAR INJURIES: TREATMENT AND OUTCOME

PETER M. MURRAY, MD

Perilunate dislocations and perilunate fracture-dislocations are the most devastating closed injuries of the wrist. Both are commonly missed on initial examination, potentially leading to devastating complications. These lesions occur as the final stage of an injury spectrum progressing around the wrist in a radial-to-ulnar direction. In patients who sustain a high-energy wrist injury, radiographs must be carefully scrutinized for a perilunate dislocation variant: the transscaphoid perilunate dislocation. This variant of perilunate dislocation is perhaps more readily identifiable as a result of the more obvious fracture of the scaphoid. Prompt open reduction and internal fixation of the scaphoid fracture with ligament repair, stabilization, or reconstruction is necessary to achieve favorable results. Posttraumatic arthrosis may result following these injuries, irrespective of treatment. Posttraumatic degenerative arthritis typically requires a salvage procedure.

Little is known about the actual incidence of perilunate dislocations and perilunate fracture-dislocations. Wrist injuries often are not appreciated, and many believe that perilunate injuries in general are underdiagnosed. Perilunate dislocation, lunate dislocation, and perilunate fracture-dislocation variants have been estimated to account for less than 10% of all wrist injuries.[1] In one study reviewing perilunate dislocations, 61% were of the transscaphoid perilunate type.[2]

ANATOMY

The carpal bones of the wrist joint are arranged in two rows: the proximal carpal row (scaphoid, lunate, and triquetrum) and the distal carpal row (trapezium, trapezoid, capitate, and hamate). The wrist joint is composed of intrinsic and extrinsic ligaments. The intrinsic ligaments are short and stout; they stabilize adjacent carpal bones. Extrinsic ligaments span either the proximal carpal row, the distal carpal row, or both.

Within the proximal carpal row, the scapholunate interosseous ligament helps to stabilize the scaphoid-lunate articulation. The scapholunate interosseous ligament has three portions: proximal, dorsal, and volar.[3] The dorsal portion of this ligament provides most of the stabilizing strength of the scapholunate articulation. The lunotriquetral interosseous ligament secures the articulation of the lunate and the triquetrum. Although stout, the interosseous ligaments of the proximal carpal row allow relative motion between the scaphoid and lunate and the lunate and the triquetrum.

The extrinsic carpal ligaments provide structural integrity for the articulations of the proximal and distal carpal rows (**Figure 1**). The radioscaphocapitate (RSC) ligament originates from the radial styloid, crosses the waist of the scaphoid, and insets on the volar waist region of the capitate. Immediately ulnar to the RSC is the radiolunotriquetral ligament, which origi-

FIGURE 1

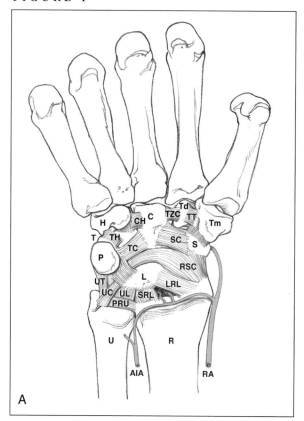

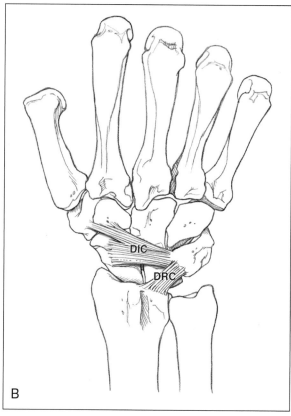

Extrinsic ligaments of the wrist. **A,** Palmar view. RA= radial artery; AIA= anterior interosseous artery; R = radius; U = ulna; PRU = proximal radioulnar ligament; UC = ulnocapitate ligament; UL = ulnolunate ligament; UT = ulnotriquetral ligament; SRL = short radiolunate ligament; P = pisiform; L = lunate; LRL = long radiolunate ligament; T = triquetrum; TH = triquetralhamate ligament; TC = triquetralcapitate ligament; RSC = radioscaphocapitate ligament; H = hamate; CH = capitohamate ligament; C = capitate; SC = scaphocapitate ligament; S = scaphoid; TZC= trapezoidalcapitate; Td = trapezoid; TT = trapezoidaltripezial ligament; Tm = trapezium. **B,** Dorsal view. DIC= dorsal intercarpal ligament; DRC = dorsal radiocarpal ligament. (Reproduced with permission from the Mayo Foundation.)

nates from the radial styloid, sends an attachment to the volar aspect of the lunate, and then terminates on the triquetrum. The short radiolunate ligament originates from the most ulnar aspect of the distal radial articular surface and inserts on the proximal volar aspect of the lunate. Two ligaments originate from the base of the ulnar styloid: the ulnocapitate and the ulnotriquetral. A portion of the ulnotriquetral ligament continues across the midcarpal joint to insert on the waist of the capitate and to join the RSC forming an inverted V. This is the *ulnocapitate ligament* and the inverted V confluence is the *arcuate ligament.* Just proximal to the base of the V is a soft spot, the space of *Porier.* Found between the

short radiolunate ligament and the radiolunotriquetral ligament is the RSL ligament, which is also called the *ligament of Testut.* The "ligament" designation is a misnomer; histologic studies have shown that this is a vascular structure devoid of any true collagen fibers and lacking any structural integrity.[3,4]

Within the dorsal capsule of the wrist are two ligaments of particular importance: the dorsal intercarpal ligament and the dorsal radiocarpal ligament. The dorsal intercarpal ligament courses transversely from the waist of the scaphoid across the carpus inserting on to the dorsal aspect of the triquetrum. The dorsal radiocarpal ligament spans from its origin on the radial styloid and inserts on the dorsal aspect of the triquetrum. Together, these two ligaments form a V with the base of the V on the triquetrum. The less substantial dorsal wrist capsule is between the limbs of the V.

WRIST BIOMECHANICS

The carpus articulates in flexion and extension as well as in radial and ulnar deviation, with synchronous motion occurring between the radiocarpal and midcarpal joints. Relatively small amounts of dynamic intracarpal supination and pronation also occur.[5] In the normal wrist, the midcarpal joint contributes 43% and the radiocarpal joint 57% of flexion and extension.[6] Linscheid and associates[7] equate the coordinated motion of the proximal and distal carpal rows as a "slider crank," like the three-bar linkage engineered to run steam locomotives. In this model, the authors describe the scaphoid as representing the crank. In the normal wrist, the scaphoid rests in approximately 45° relative to the long axis of the forearm and is susceptible to injury. The triquetrum has a helicoid articulation with the hamate that creates potential energy for triquetral extension; the position of the scaphoid creates potential energy for flexion.[8] As a result, the lunate is dynamically balanced from the energy transferred through the scapholunate interosseous and the lunotriquetral interosseous ligaments. In radial deviation, the distal carpal row inclines toward the radial styloid, and the proximal carpal row shifts toward the ulna. For radial deviation to progress, the scaphoid must flex beyond 45° to avoid radial-styloid impingement. The result is relative flexion of the entire proximal row to accomplish radial deviation of the wrist.[8] In a reciprocal fashion, ulnar deviation causes the distal carpal row to shift toward the ulna and the proximal carpal row translates toward the radial styloid. Because of the helicoid articulation of the triquetrum with the hamate, the proximal carpal row extends with ulnar deviation of the wrist.[8] The carpal height measured from the distal articular surface of the radius to the base of the third metacarpal remains constant throughout the limits of radial and ulnar deviation and wrist flexion and extension.[9] Short, stout ligaments between the bones of the distal carpal row permit only negligible amounts of hamate-capitate intracarpal motion.[10]

FIGURE 2

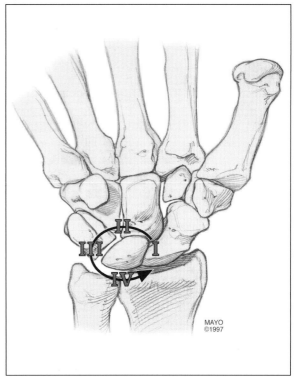

Staged progression of the perilunar injury of the wrist as described by Mayfied. Stage I= Scapholunate dissociation; stage II= Capitolunate (injury through space of Poirier); stage III= Lunotriquetral dissociation; stage IV= Disruption of the short and long radiolunate ligaments. (Reproduced with permission from the Mayo Foundation.)

MECHANISM OF INJURY

Young adults experience high-energy, transscaphoid perilunate dislocations of the wrist, often the result of falling from a height or a motor vehicle accident; the pronated forearm locks an outstretched wrist that is axially loaded, ulnarly deviated, and extended beyond 100°. The ultimate impact position of the wrist likely determines the type of perilunar variant injury.

Mayfield and colleagues,[11] in a cadaver model, were able to recreate perilunate and lunate dislocations in the laboratory. By mounting cadaver arms vertically and applying a radial-to-ulnar directed force with wrist extension and intracarpal supination, perilunate and lunate dislocations were created following four distinct stages (**Figure 2**). In stage 1, the scapholunate interosseous and the radioscaphocapitate ligament ruptured. In the transscaphoid variant, the injury force is transmitted through the scaphoid instead of the scapholunate interosseous ligament (SLIL) and the radioscaphocapitate ligament. Following scaphoid fracture, the injury progresses through the space of Poirer during the second stage of the injury. In the third stage, rupture of the lunotriquetral interosseous ligament occurs. The failure of the lunotriquetral interosseous ligament permits the perilunate aspect of the injury and enables such lesions as the transscaphoid perilunate dislocation. In stage four, the short and long radiolunate ligaments are disrupted, permitting dislocation of the lunate.

Diagnosis

Perilunate dislocations, including transscaphoid perilunate dislocations, are diagnosed late in up to 25% of patients.[2] Patients with a wrist dislocation variant generally present with deformity, swelling, and pain. However, in any patient presenting with wrist pain after high-energy wrist trauma, a wrist dislocation or variant should be suspected. A careful trauma assessment is mandatory, including careful examination for associated injuries to the head, thorax, pelvis, and other extremities. Careful inspection of the wrist is imperative to rule out an open injury. Vascular and neurologic examinations are performed, being mindful that median nerve injury often may be associated with transscaphoid perilunate dislocation of the wrist.

Standard posteroanterior (PA) and lateral radiographs are obtained after removal of any splint material and dressings. Acute distraction or traction views of the carpus may better define the injury, specifically helping to identify associated carpal fractures. The PA view is inspected for disruption of the lines of Gilula (**Figure 3, A** and *B*). These lines can be traced along the proximal articular surfaces of the scaphoid, lunate, and triquetrum, as well as the proximal surfaces of the trapezium, trapezoid, capitate, and hamate. Any disruption of the otherwise smooth contour of these lines should be considered diagnostic of intracarpal derangement. Alternatively, the lateral view of the carpus should be carefully viewed for the fat carpus sign (**Figure 3**, *C*). The fat carpus sign in a dorsal perilunate dislocation or perilunate dislocation variant occurs when the capitate

and the remainder of the carpus are dorsal to and over-riding the lunate.

In most situations, plain radiography with or without distraction views is sufficient to diagnose the transscaphoid perilunate dislocation. CT or plain tomography may be necessary to identify associated fractures that may occur as a result of greater arch injuries of the carpus.

Injury Classification

When considered in the broader scheme of wrist instability, transscaphoid perilunate fracture-dislocations of the wrist reside in the category carpal instability complex (**Table 1**). In carpal instability complex, there are elements of both dissociative and nondissociative carpal instability. Failure of the lunotriquetral interosseous ligament accounts for the dissociative instability component and disruption of the midcarpal articulation accounts for the nondissociative component.

Based on their clinical experiences, Green and O'Brien[12] developed a classification system for perilunate dislocations and their variants (**Table 2**). The most common pure perilunate dislocation is the dorsal dislocation, and the most common lunate dislocation is the volar lunate dislocation. In one review of perilunate dislocations,[2] 61% were of the transscaphoid perilunate variety, which are considered the most common wrist dislocation. Included in their classification system is the exceptionally rare pure greater arc injury or the transscaphoid, transcapitate, transtriquetral perilunate fracture pattern (type IV B).

Treatment

Acute transscaphoid perilunate fracture-dislocations or other wrist dislocations require prompt reduction. Because the carpus generally dislocates dorsally in these injuries, prompt reduction is essential to protect the median nerve. Volar transscaphoid perilunate dislocations also have been described.[13] Reduction of the wrist is facilitated by emergent transfer to the operating room where the procedure can be performed under regional or general anesthesia. Treatment of life- or limb-threatening injuries must take precedence, possibly delaying or postponing open reduction and internal fixation of the scaphoid fracture and soft-tissue repair or recon-

FIGURE 3

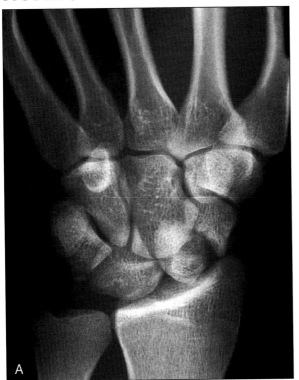

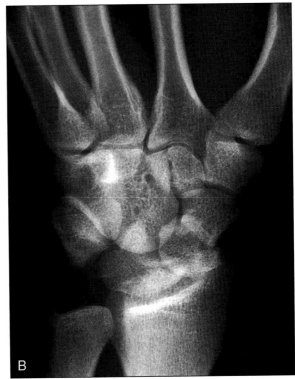

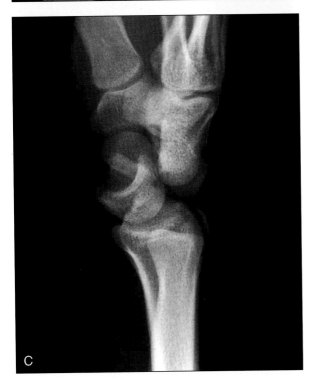

PA **(A)**, oblique **(B)**, and lateral **(C)** radiographs of a transscaphoid dorsal perilunate dislocation of the wrist demonstrating the disruption of the smooth line of Gilula along proximal articular surfaces of the scaphoid, lunate, and triquetrum. (Reproduced with permission from the Mayo Foundation.)

TABLE 1

Mayo Classification of Carpal Instability

Dissociative Carpal Instability (CID)
Proximal carpal row
Unstable scaphoid fracture
Scapholunate dissociation
Lunotriquetral dissociation

Distal carpal row
Axial radial disruption
Axial ulnar disruption
Combined

Combined proximal and distal carpal rows

Nondissociative Carpal Instability (CIND)
Radiocarpal
Palmar ligament rupture
Dorsal ligament rupture
After "radius malunion," Madelung's deformity, scaphoid
    malunion, lunate malunion (See adaptive carpus below.)

Midcarpal
Ulnar midcarpal instability from palmar ligament damage
Radial midcarpal instability from palmar ligament damage
Combined ulnar and radial midcarpal instability, palmar
    ligament damage
Midcarpal instability from dorsal ligament damage

Combined radiocarpal-midcarpal
Capitolunate instability pattern (CLIP)
Disruption of radial and central ligaments

Carpal Instability Complex (CIC)
Perilunate with radiocarpal instability
Perilunate with axial instability
Radiocarpal with axial instability
Scapholunate dissociation with ulnar translation

Adaptive Carpal Instability (CIA)
Malposition of carpus with distal radius malunion
Malposition of carpus with scaphoid nonunion
Malposition of carpus with lunate malunion
Malposition of carpus with Madelung's deformity

(Reproduced with permission from Dobyns JH, Cooney WP:
Classification of carpal instability, in Cooney WP, Linscheid RL,
Dobyns JH (eds): *The Wrist: Diagnosis and Surgical Treatment.*
St. Louis, MO, Mosby, 1998, pp 490-500.)

TABLE 2

Classification of Carpal Dislocations

Type	Description
I	Dorsal perilunate/volar lunate dislocation
II	Dorsal transscaphoid perilunate dislocation
III	Volar perilunate/dorsal lunate dislocation
IV	Variants
	A Transradial styloid perilunate dislocation
	B Naviculocapitate syndrome
	C Transtriquetral fracture-dislocation
	D Miscellaneous
V	Isolated rotary scaphoid subluxation
	A Acute subluxation
	B Recurrent subluxation
VI	Total dislocation of the scaphoid

(Reproduced with permission from Green DP, O'Brien ET:
Classification and management of carpal dislocation. *Clin
Orthop* 1980: 149;55-72.)

---

made unless contraindicated by soft-tissue swelling. Regardless of the clinical situation, reduction of the dislocation must proceed urgently.

To obtain initial closed reduction of the transscaphoid perilunate dislocation, the wrist is hyperextended and distracted. Counterpressure is applied to the volar aspect of the wrist joint, and the head of the capitate is engaged into the distal fossa of the lunate. The wrist is then volarly flexed to complete the reduction. If associated injuries or conditions delay transfer to the operating room, the initial reduction may be attempted in the emergency department under conscious sedation and local anesthesia. Closed reduction may be facilitated by 5 to 7 minutes of initial finger trap traction applied with 10 to 15 lb of weight.

Definitive fixation of the scaphoid is accomplished with the palmar approach for midwaist fractures or through the dorsal approach for fractures involving the proximal pole. The dorsal approach also is necessary under circumstances when rupture of the SLIL is suspected. Rupture of the SLIL rarely occurs in association with a transscaphoid, perilunate dislocation. Scaphoid and lunate relationships also may be difficult to assess with radiographs of the acute transscaphoid perilunate dislocation of the wrist. Once initial emergent closed or open radiocarpal and midcarpal joint reduction is performed, a distraction view or an ulnar deviation view

struction. Although internal fixation and soft-tissue repair or reconstruction can be delayed after reduction of the wrist dislocation, promptly proceeding with definitive treatment is recommended once the diagnosis is

FIGURE 4

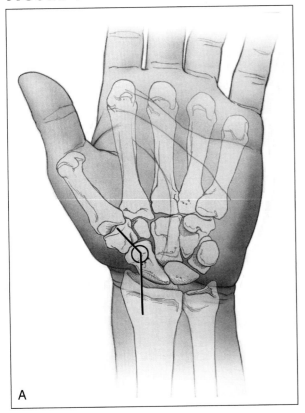
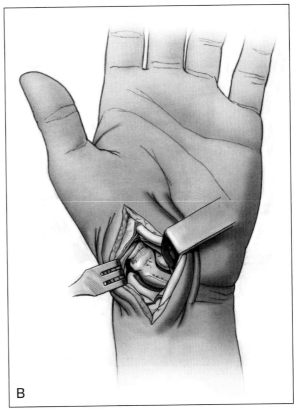

A, An angled incision is used to approach the volar scaphoid with the apex of the incision over the volar scaphoid tuberosity. **B,** Once the approach is made (through the floor of the FCR sheath and by dividing the long radiolunate and radioscaphocapitate ligaments), the scaphoid waist and distal pole can be readily evaluated. (Reproduced with permission from the Mayo Foundation.)

of the carpus may help to define the integrity of the SLIL.

PALMAR APPROACH

The palmar approach is most commonly used for scaphoid fixation. An inverted L incision is preferred (**Figure 4**, *A*), and the sheath of the flexor carpi radialis (FCR) tendon is incised. The distal aspect of the incision is extended along the thenar eminence where the glabrous skin meets the skin of the dorsum of the thumb. The FCR tendon, along with the palmar cutaneous branch of the median nerve, are retracted ulnarly. The floor of the FCR sheath is then incised, followed by incision of the volar radial wrist capsule (**Figure 4**, *B*). Care is exercised to preserve as much of the RSC liga-

ment as possible. The scaphoid is reduced with Kirschner wire (K-wire) joy sticks or by the use of external instrumentation. Once reduced, a longitudinal K-wire is used to secure the reduction. A small volar portion of the trapezium is removed to facilitate placement of a cannulated compression screw. Failure to osteotomize the trapezium may result in suboptimal dorsal placement of the compression screw.[14] Compression screw placement through the volar approach is detailed in a separate chapter.

Once acceptable reduction has been obtained, the volar wrist capsule is closed. It is my practice to proceed with a prophylactic carpal tunnel release through a separate incision that crosses the wrist. Also through this incision the full extent of the volar wrist capsule may be inspected and any transverse defect may be repaired. For comminuted waist scaphoid fractures with marked displacement or humpback deformity, a volar wedge bone graft may be necessary to adequately stabilize the fracture reduction construct. Once satisfactory reduction and stabilization have been achieved, the volar wrist capsule is closed with interrupted bioabsorbable sutures. This is followed by a layered closure for the subcutaneous layers and the skin.

DORSAL APPROACH

For fractures involving the proximal scaphoid pole, the dorsal approach is preferred. The dorsal approach is safe as long as the blood supply along the distal dorsal radial aspect of the scaphoid is protected during the surgical exposure. A longitudinal incision is made just proximal to Lister's tubercle and extended just beyond the midcarpal joint. The third dorsal compartment is incised, and the extensor pollicis longus tendon is delivered out of the compartment and retracted radially. The fourth dorsal compartment is then elevated subperiosteally and ulnarly to expose the dorsal wrist capsule. The dorsal wrist capsule consists of the dorsal radial triquetral ligament and the dorsal radiocarpal ligament. The triangular portion of capsule between these two ligaments can be raised with a radially based flap exposing the proximal pole of the scaphoid and the SLIL. The dorsal exposure facilitates open reduction and internal fixation of the proximal pole fracture beyond that which can be obtained through the palmar approach. Hyperflexion of the wrist can assist in placement of a cannulated compression screw for proximal scaphoid fractures. Further details of dorsal approach compression screw placement for proximal pole scaphoid fractures is found in a separate chapter.

Once secure fixation is obtained for the scaphoid fracture, the SLIL must be inspected for rupture. Direct repair of the ligament is preferred, provided that the ligament is of sufficient quality. Before reducing the scapholunate interosseous interval, it is desirable to first place sutures for repair. The SLIL more commonly avulses from the scaphoid proximal pole, which will accept two or three suture anchors with No. 4-0 braided, nonabsorbable suture. Infrequently, the SLIL detaches from the lunate. An alternative technique requires drill holes placed in the scaphoid pole, exiting along the radial ridge of the scaphoid.[15] In this technique, braided No.

4-0 nonabsorbable sutures are passed through the SLIL then through the scaphoid, reapproximating the SLIL to the scaphoid.

Whatever technique is chosen, the sutures should be passed before the scapholunate interval is reduced and a small area of subchondral bone exposed for reattachment of the SLIL. The internally fixed scaphoid is then reduced to the lunate by stabilizing the lunate and extending the wrist until the desired lateral scapholunate angle is achieved. The lateral scapholunate angle is assessed by using intraoperative fluoroscopy, with the normal lateral scapholunate angle ranging between 30° and 60°.[7] Once the desired angle is achieved, a 0.045-in K-wire is advanced from the scaphoid into the lunate. An additional 0.045-in K-wire is then advanced from the scaphoid waist region into the body of the capitate. K-wire placement in the distal pole of the scaphoid is avoided because the volar flexed position of the scaphoid does not align with the capitate. The previously placed suture is then secured, advancing the SLIL to its previous site of insertion.

Ideally, the lunotriquetral interosseous ligament should be repaired as well. This, however, is technically difficult because of the tight articulation between the lunate and the triquetrum. In most circumstances, the lunotriquetral interval can be adequately stabilized with one or two 0.045 in K-wires placed from the triquetrum into the lunate. I currently augment any SLIL repair with a dorsal capsulodesis, regardless of the integrity of the ligament. A variety of capsulodesis techniques have been described. One approach is to detach the triquetral insertion of the dorsal intercarpal ligament, rotating it and securing it to the dorsum of the lunate (RA Berger, MD, PhD, personal communication, 2006). This seems to have the biomechanical advantage of applying a compressive force to the scapholunate articulation and the practical advantage of not crossing the radiocarpal joint. These theoretical advantages, however, have not been studied biomechanically.

POSTOPERATIVE REHABILITATION

The greatest shortcoming in the current management of transscaphoid perilunate dislocation of the wrist is the prolonged period of wrist immobilization necessary to ensure healing of the scaphoid and wrist ligaments. Early efforts to restore motion and strength can cause

FIGURE 5

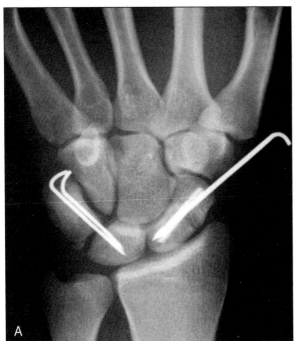 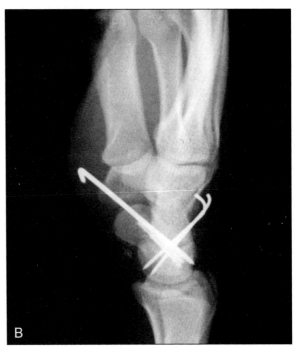

Postoperative PA **(A)** and lateral **(B)** radiographs of a transscaphoid perilunate dislocation demonstrating internal fixation of the scaphoid and K-wire stabilization of the lunotriquetral joint after ligament repair. (Reproduced with permission from the Mayo Foundation.)

failure of bony as well as soft-tissue healing. Thumb spica cast immobilization is necessary after open reduction and internal fixation of transscaphoid perilunate wrist dislocations. Alternatively, external fixation of the wrist also has been advocated.

Following wound closure, a bulky dressing, a forearm-based thumb spica plaster dressing, and a commercially available arm cooling device are applied. During the ensuing 72 hours, the patient is instructed on strict arm elevation. Hospital discharge instructions include directions on digital motion and measures to prevent swelling. On postoperative day 2, the wound is examined and the dressing reapplied, applying another forearm-based thumb spica splint, which is maintained for approximately 2 weeks. At 2 weeks postoperatively, the sutures are removed and a short arm thumb spica cast applied. This cast is maintained for 12 weeks. During this phase of rehabilitation, the patient is seen regularly by a hand therapist and instructed on finger motion and on measures to prevent swelling of the fingers. Overhead fisting maneuvers provide another method of con-

trolling finger swelling and preventing adhesive capsulitis of the shoulder. Active and passive elbow motion also is encouraged. Activities of daily living are incorporated into the first phase of the rehabilitation of wrist dislocations for both therapeutic and functional reasons. PA and lateral radiographs are obtained at 2 and 6 weeks postoperatively to ensure continued reduction of the midcarpal and radiocarpal joints (**Figure 5**). PA, lateral, and scaphoid views of the wrist are obtained at 3 months to assess scaphoid healing. I order CT of the scaphoid at 3 months postoperatively if there is any question about scaphoid healing.

At 12 weeks postoperatively, the cast or external fixator is removed and the patient is converted to a removable, custom-molded, forearm-based thumb spica splint. Under the direction of a hand therapist, the patient removes the splint daily to perform gentle active range-of-motion exercises. Following periods of prolonged immobilization, profound forearm weakness is expected. Neuromuscular reeducation is necessary to overcome compensatory movements such as co-contraction.

Ultrasound and superficial heating agents can be used to reduce pain and facilitate range of motion.

At 18 weeks postoperatively and once scaphoid healing is confirmed, more aggressive rehabilitation is initiated, including passive and active-assist wrist motion. Although limited range of motion goals exist following these injuries, dynamic flexion and extension splinting for the wrist can be used for particularly recalcitrant cases. Static splinting is discontinued at this time, and resistance strengthening is delayed until 6 months postoperatively. Delays in scaphoid union delays this portion of the rehabilitation regime. A frank discussion with the patient is necessary so that it is understood that the limitations in range of motion and strength deficits are likely permanent.

Chronic Injuries

The diagnosis and management of many wrist dislocations and fracture-dislocations often are delayed, which adversely affects outcomes.[16,17] Patients with undiagnosed perilunate or lunate dislocations present with nonremitting wrist pain, limited motion, deformity, or median nerve symptoms.

Appropriate treatment options include late open reduction and internal fixation of the scaphoid with ligamentous reconstruction as indicated, proximal row carpectomy, limited wrist arthrodesis, or complete wrist arthrodesis. Open reduction and internal fixation for chronic transscaphoid perilunate dislocations should be considered first. Gradual distraction using external fixation or ring fixation can be considered to address soft-tissue contracture. It has been my experience that, with aggressive postoperative physical therapy after open reduction of chronic wrist locations of up to 3 months, the digital extension lag resulting from tendon and muscle contracture can be overcome. Inoue and Shionoya[18] reported three good, one fair, and two poor results in six patients with chronic transscaphoid dorsal perilunate dislocations treated with open reduction and internal fixation at an average of 16 weeks after injury.

In patients with long-standing transscaphoid perilunate dislocations, restoration of length can cause median nerve or even vascular dysfunction. For patients in whom direct reduction and internal fixation are not feasible, salvage techniques can be performed with predictable results. Rettig and Raskin[19] reported good results in 12 patients with chronic perilunate dislocation or dislocation variants, treated by proximal row carpectomy at an average of 40 months follow-up. Their patients noted pain relief, improved motion, and enhanced grip strength. In patients with articular defects, limited arthrodesis (such as scaphoidectomy and four-corner fusion) or complete wrist arthrodesis should be considered.

Complications

Posttraumatic arthritis generally is recognized as the most common complication following either acute or late treatment of transscaphoid perilunate dislocations of the wrist.[13] Separate studies have identified posttraumatic arthritis following acute management of perilunate fracture-dislocations in more than 50% of patients.[13,20] Wrist stiffness and loss of grip strength are also expected complications.[20] Also recognized is median nerve dysfunction after all perilunate fracture-dislocations, particularly chronically unreduced dislocations.[16] Late presentation of median nerve paresthesias has been reported more than 60 years after an unreduced dorsal perilunate dislocation.[17] Late carpal instability is a recognized complication after perilunate fracture-dislocations and is regarded as particularly difficult to manage.[21] Residual carpal instability in these patients may be scapholunate instability (dissociative carpal instability if injury of the SLIL has occurred), ulnar translation of the carpus (nondissociative carpal instability), or midcarpal instability (nondissociative carpal instability).

Osteonecrosis of the scaphoid and the lunate also is a potential complication following transscaphoid perilunate fracture-dislocations. Osteonecrosis of the lunate is rare and should not be confused with transient ischemia as described by White and Omer.[22] Scaphoid nonunion may be seen as a complication and is more likely when adequate scaphoid stabilization has not been achieved. Theoretically, scaphoid nonunion seems more common in the setting of a transscaphoid perilunate fracture-dislocation than in the isolated scaphoid fracture because of the associated wrist instability of the perilunate injury. This circumstance, however, has never been satisfactorily shown.

OUTCOMES

When left untreated, the results of transscaphoid perilunate dislocations are poor because of the combination of loss of motion, pain, and median nerve dysfunction.[16] It has been reported that anywhere from 25% to 33% of all perilunate dislocations, including the transscaphoid variant, are initially missed.[13,16] Despite treatment within 1 week, Herzberg and associates[2] showed that posttraumatic arthritis develops in 56% of patients. In this multicenter review, 115 patients were followed 6 years; treatment delays and open injuries correlated with poor results. Better results were obtained in patients who underwent open reduction and internal fixation compared with those who had closed reduction and percutaneous pinning. In another study, 14 transscaphoid perilunate dislocations were evaluated at an average of 8 years postoperatively.[23] Surgery was performed an average of 6 days after injury. Thirteen patients underwent open reduction and internal fixation, whereas one patient underwent a proximal row carpectomy. The average Mayo wrist score was 79%, and all scaphoid fractures internally fixed healed. Posttraumatic arthritis was observed radiographically in all patients. Limited return of range of motion and strength can be expected.

CONCLUSIONS

Transscaphoid perilunate dislocations of the wrist are unusual, high-energy injuries of the wrist that require prompt treatment. Up to 33% of perilunate fracture-dislocations of all types are initially missed and come to treatment late. The transscaphoid dorsal perilunate dislocation comprises 61% of all perilunate fracture-dislocations.[2] Considered in a broader sense, the transscaphoid perilunate fracture-dislocation is the end result of a four-stage injury that progresses through the carpus in a radial-to-ulnar direction.[11] Physical examination of patients suspected of having a transscaphoid perilunate fracture-dislocation requires careful inspection of the skin and a detailed neurologic examination. The diagnosis generally can be made using standard PA and lateral radiographs. Accurate open reduction of the scaphoid is necessary with repair of the SLIL, if injured, as well as volar extrinsic capsular ligaments. After surgery, immobilization is typically prolonged because of the extended time necessary to ensure scaphoid fracture

and ligamentous healing. Although often suggested, the incidence of scaphoid nonunion in the setting of transscaphoid perilunate dislocation is no greater than the incidence of nonunion in isolated scaphoid fractures.[24] After appropriate management of wrist dislocations, a functional wrist with diminished motion and strength can be expected.

Complications of perilunate dislocations generally include posttraumatic arthritis, chronic pain, and median nerve dysfunction. In some situations, treatment still can be successful in chronic untreated transscaphoid perilunate dislocations, but salvage reconstructive procedures such as proximal row carpectomy, scaphoidectomy, four-corner fusion, or complete wrist arthrodesis are often necessary. In general, better results generally can be expected with early surgical intervention, focusing on acute joint reduction, fractures reduction, and ligamentous repair as needed.

REFERENCES

1. Minami A, Kaneda K: Repair and/or reconstruction of scapholunate interosseous ligament in lunate and perilunate dislocations. *J Hand Surg [Am]* 1993;18:1099-1106.

2. Berger RA: The gross and histologic anatomy of the scapholunate interosseous ligament. *J Hand Surg [Am]* 1996;21:170-178.

3. Berger RA, Kauer JM, Landsmeer JM: Radioscapholunate ligament: A gross anatomic and histologic study of fetal and adult wrists. *J Hand Surg [Am]* 1991;16:350-355.

4. Kobayashi M, Berger RA, Linscheid RL, An KN: Intercarpal kinematics during wrist motion. *Hand Clin* 1997;13:143-149.

5. Wolfe SW, Crisco JJ, Katz LD: A non-invasive method for studying in vivo carpal kinematics. *J Hand Surg [Br]* 1997;22:147-152.

6. Linscheid RL, Dobyns JH, Beabout JW, Bryan RS: Traumatic instability of the wrist. Diagnosis, classification, and pathomechanics. *J Bone Joint Surg Am* 1972;54:1612-1632.

7. Shin A, Murray P: Biomechanical studies of wrist ligament injuries, in Trumble T (ed): *Carpal Fracture-Dislocations*. Chicago, IL, American Academy of Orthopaedic Surgeons, 2002, pp 7-18.

8. Youm Y, McMurthy RY, Flatt AE, Gillespie TE: Kinematics of the wrist. I. An experimental study of radial-ulnar deviation and flexion-extension. *J Bone Joint Surg Am* 1978;60:423-431.

9. Ritt MJ, Berger RA, Bishop AT, An KN: The capitohamate ligaments. A comparison of biomechanical properties. *J Hand Surg [Br]* 1996;21:451-454.

10. Mayfield JK, Johnson RP, Kilcoyne RK: Carpal dislocations: Pathomechanics and progressive perilunar instability. *J Hand Surg Am* 1980;5:226-241.

11. Herzberg G, Comtet JJ, Linscheid RL, Amadio PC, Cooney WP, Stalder J: Perilunate dislocations and fracture-dislocations: a multicenter study. *J Hand Surg [Am]* 1993;18:768-779.

12. Green DP, O'Brien ET: Classification and management of carpal dislocations. *Clin Orthop Relat Res* 1980;149:55-72.

13. Carmichael KD, Bell C: Volar perilunate trans-scaphoid fracture-dislocation in a skeletally immature patient. *Orthopedics* 2005;28:69-70.

14. Trumble TE, Clarke T, Kreder HJ: Non-union of the scaphoid. Treatment with cannulated screws compared with treatment with Herbert screws. *J Bone Joint Surg Am* 1996;78:1829-1837.

15. Taleisnik J, Linscheid R: Scapholunate instability, in Cooney WP, Linscheid RL, Dobyns JH (eds): *The Wrist: Diagnosis and Operative Treatment*. St. Louis, MO, Mosby, 1998, pp 490-500.

16. Campbell RD Jr, Lance EM, Yeoh CB: Lunate and perilunar dislocations. *J Bone Joint Surg Br* 1964;46:55-72.

17. Tomaino MM: Late management of perilunate fracture-dislocations, in Trumble T (ed): *Carpal Fracture-Dislocations*. Chicago, IL, American Academy of Orthopaedic Surgeons, 2002, pp 7-18.

18. Inoue G, Shionoya K: Late treatment of unreduced perilunate dislocations. *J Hand Surg [Br]* 1999;24:221-225.

19. Rettig ME, Raskin KB: Long-term assessment of proximal row carpectomy for chronic perilunate dislocations. *J Hand Surg [Am]* 1999;24:1231-1236.

20. Sotereanos DG, Mitsionis GJ, Giannakopoulos PN, Tomaino MM, Herndon JH: Perilunate dislocation and fracture dislocation: a critical analysis of the volar-dorsal approach. *J Hand Surg [Am]* 1997;22:49-56.

21. Kozin SH, Murphy M, Cooney W: Perilunate dislocations, in Cooney WP, Linscheid RL, Dobyns JH (eds): *The Wrist: Diagnosis and Operative Treatment*. St. Louis, MO, Mosby, 1998, pp 632-650.

22. White RE Jr, Omer GE Jr: Transient vascular compromise of the lunate after fracture-dislocation or dislocation of the carpus. *J Hand Surg [Am]* 1984;9:181-184.

23. Herzberg G, Forissier D: Acute dorsal trans-scaphoid perilunate fracture-dislocations: medium-term results. *J Hand Surg [Br]* 2002;27:498-502.

24. Murray PM: Dislocations of the wrist: Carpal instability complex. *J Am Soc Surg Hand* 2003;3:88-99.

CHAPTER 7

SCAPHOID FRACTURES IN CHILDREN

BASSEM T. ELHASSAN, MD
ALEXANDER Y. SHIN, MD
SCOTT H. KOZIN, MD

Carpal fractures are uncommon in children.[1] However, scaphoid fractures are the most commonly fractured carpal bone, accounting for 3% of all fractures of the hand and wrist and 0.45% of all fractures in the upper limb in children.[2-5] A scaphoid fracture in a child with open physeal growth plates is considered a pediatric scaphoid fracture. Scaphoid fractures have a peak incidence between the ages of 12 and 15 years.[2-4,6-9] Few reported cases involve children younger than 8 years of age; the youngest patient reported is 4 years of age.[1,10-13]

The low incidence of scaphoid fractures in children is most likely related to the thick peripheral cartilage that covers and protects the ossification center. Therefore, considerable force is required to disrupt this cartilaginous shell and injure the underlying bone.[14] The pattern of pediatric scaphoid injury in children differs from that of adults because of the evolving changes in the ossification center.[5,15,16] During early stages of ossification, the scaphoid is more susceptible to avulsion fractures about the distal pole fracture.[1,17] Ossification progresses from distal to proximal, and the fracture pattern mirrors the adult forms by early adolescence. This chapter reviews the development, mechanism of injury, associated injuries, diagnosis, classification, and treatment options of pediatric scaphoid fractures.

SCAPHOID DEVELOPMENT

Normal Development

The cartilaginous model present in utero expands in size during prenatal and postnatal development. The ossific nucleus of the scaphoid appears at approximately 5 years and 10 months of age in boys and 4 years and 6 months of age in girls.[10,18] Multiple ossification centers occasionally may appear, but coalescence is rapid.[11] Initially, the scaphoid is composed of articular cartilage that covers extensive epiphyseal cartilage, which progressively undergoes enchondral ossification.[7] Enchondral ossification forms about the distal aspect and grows in an eccentric mode until ossification is complete, by the age of 15 years in boys and 13.5 years in girls. The cartilaginous model of the scaphoid is completely ossified by skeletal maturity. The only remaining cartilage covers the articular surface. This chondro-osseous transformation depends on local perfusion supplied by the extensive blood supply occupying the cartilage canal system.[2]

Variations

The topic of a bipartite scaphoid continues to be controversial. In support of this concept, Gruber[19] and Pfitzner[20] found four specimens among 3,007 dissections, and later Pfitzner[21] noted nine cases in 1,450 anatomic studies. These authors proposed that scaphoid bipartition is an infrequent developmental variation that results from failure of fusion of the proximal ulnar and the distal radial components of the scaphoid.[5] In contrast, Louis and colleagues[22] believe that bipartition of the scaphoid does not exist but represents a previously undiagnosed injury. Their dissections of 196 human fetuses (gestational age ranging from 4 to 30 weeks) failed to identify any bipartite scaphoids. These authors also reviewed hand radiographs of 11,280 children and were unable to find a single instance of bipartite scaphoid.

MECHANISM OF INJURY

The most common mechanism of scaphoid fracture is a fall onto the outstretched hand and pronated forearm, which exerts tensile forces acting across the volar portion of the scaphoid.[23] In children, there are other potential causes related to their specific activities. Toh and associates[24] reviewed 64 scaphoid fractures in children between the ages of 11 and 15 years. The most common mechanism of injury was sporting activities in 27 patients, punching game machines or fighting in 22, and motor vehicle accidents or other trauma in 15. The most common sporting activities that cause scaphoid fractures in children are skateboarding and bicycling.[1,17]

Minor trauma can be the cause of scaphoid fracture associated with a pathologic process. Scaphoid fracture can be the initial manifestation of a patient with a scaphoid enchondroma.[25] Of the nine patients with scaphoid enchondroma reported in the literature, six presented a scaphoid fracture after minor injury.[26-30]

ASSOCIATED INJURIES

Associated injuries within the wrist or along the arm may accompany a pediatric scaphoid fracture. Associated carpal injuries include capitate fracture (also called scaphocapitate syndrome),[31-34] transscaphoid perilunate dislocation,[35,36] and other carpal fractures.[7,37] Associated limb injuries include supracondylar fracture,[38,39] distal radius fracture,[5,40-42] and metacarpal fractures.[11]

Associated injuries may be more common in younger patients. Thicker cartilage covers the bony ossification center in younger children, which renders the bone more resilient to fracture. Therefore, higher energy trauma is required to fracture the underlying scaphoid, especially in children younger than 10 years of age.[11,40,43,44]

DIAGNOSIS

The relative infrequency of this injury and the difficulty in interpreting radiographs of the immature wrist increase the rate of missing a pediatric scaphoid fracture.[1,3] The clinical presentation of a child with scaphoid fracture varies with the location of injury. A distal pole fracture presents with swelling or tenderness over the scaphoid tuberosity. A scaphoid waist fracture presents with pain to palpation within the anatomic snuffbox. Pain during axial loading of the thumb ray (painful scaphoid compression test) is suggestive of a scaphoid fracture.[45] Posteroanterior (PA), lateral, and oblique radiographs are obtained. In addition, a scaphoid view that consists of an AP view with the wrist in mild supination and the fingers flexed enhances visualization of the scaphoid. This view places the scaphoid parallel to the x-ray film and reveals the scaphoid in its full size.[46]

The physician interpreting the radiographs should be aware of the pseudo Terry-Thomas sign.[47] The scaphoid ossifies from distal to proximal, which changes the distance between the ossified lunate and scaphoid as the child approaches adolescence. This produces an increased distance between the scaphoid and lunate in the immature patient, which ranges from 9 mm in a 7-year-old child to 3 mm in a 15-year-old. Failure to appreciate these normal radiographic variants may lead to an erroneous diagnosis of scapholunate dissociation when the apparent gap is filled with normal cartilage and unossified bone. Comparison with contralateral wrist radiographs is extremely useful in distinguishing abnormal from normal patterns; however, note that carpal ossification is not always symmetric. A notch on indentation on the radial side of the scaphoid is a normal variation that is seen in approximately one third of patients.[48]

If the clinical picture is consistent with a scaphoid fracture but the radiographs are negative, the patient should be immobilized. The child should be either instructed to return in 2 weeks for a second examination and radiographs or advanced imaging studies may be ordered. MRI is useful in detecting scaphoid fractures that are not visualized on the initial radiographs

FIGURE 1

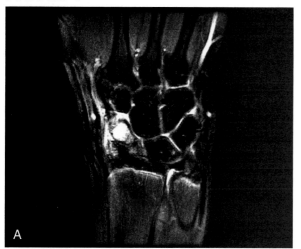 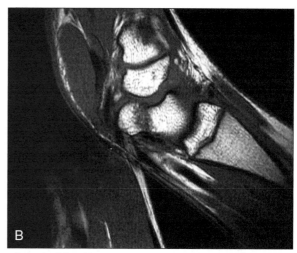

A 12-year-old boy has a 3-week history of pain in the right wrist that started after he fell on his outstretched hand. Plain radiographs were normal. Coronal T2-weighted **(A)** and sagittal T1-weighted **(B)** images of the right wrist show a fracture through the waist of scaphoid with bony edema. (Reproduced with permission from the Mayo Foundation.)

(**Figure 1**).[49,50] Johnson and co-workers[51] evaluated MRI scans of 56 children (57 injuries) within 10 days of injury. All children had a suspected scaphoid injury but normal radiographs. In 33 (58%) of the 57 injuries, the MRI scan was normal and the patients discharged. In 16 patients (28%), a fractured scaphoid was diagnosed and treatment initiated. Other fractures and abnormalities (eg, ganglion cysts) also were demonstrated on MRI. However, MRI does have drawbacks that prohibit routine use. Sedation is required in young children, and MRI may be overly sensitive in identifying bone edema that never progresses to a fracture.

Other advanced imaging studies, such as bone scans, CT, and ultrasound, also have been shown to be effective in detecting scaphoid fractures.[52-55] The role of bone scan has been nearly supplanted by MRI. In the assessment of scaphoid fracture displacement and in the determination of scaphoid union, CT is the most valuable (**Figure 2**).

CLASSIFICATION

Classification of scaphoid fractures in children is based on the stage of ossification and radiographic features (**Figure 3**).[56] A type I fracture is a pure chondral injury that occurs in children younger than 8 years. This frac-

FIGURE 2

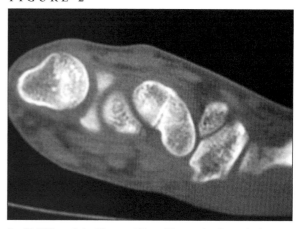

Sagittal CT scan of a 16-year-old boy with normal radiographs but persistent pain shows a nondisplaced scaphoid waist fracture. (Courtesy of Shriners Hospital for Children, Philadelphia, PA.)

ture is difficult to diagnose and requires MRI to visualize the chondral injury. A type II fracture is an osteochondral fracture that occurs in children between the ages of 8 and 11 years. A type III fracture occurs in children older than 12 years of age after the ossification center is well developed and the scaphoid bone is almost completely ossified. This is the most common type of

FIGURE 3

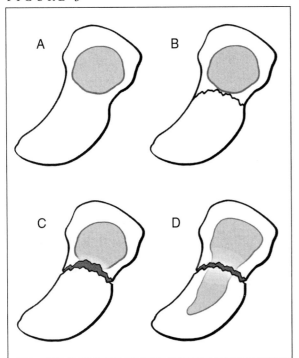

Classification of immature scaphoid. A = Normal scaphoid. B = Type I fracture: pure chondral injury. C = Type II fracture: osteochondral fracture. D = Type III fracture: adult variant fracture when the bone is nearly completely ossified. (Reproduced with permission from the Mayo Foundation.)

FIGURE 4

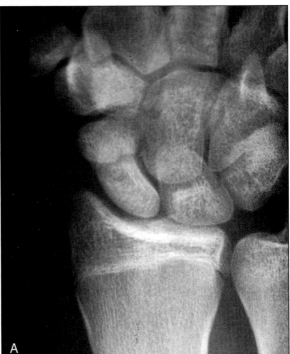

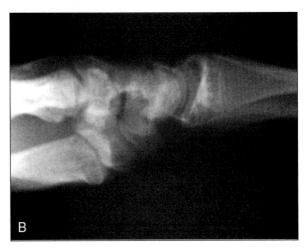

PA **(A)** and lateral **(B)** radiographs of a 14-year-old boy with a distal third scaphoid fracture. (Courtesy of Shriners Hospital for Children, Philadelphia, PA.)

scaphoid fracture in children. Each of these types of scaphoid fractures may involve any part of the scaphoid. However, the most common location in children is the distal third scaphoid fracture (**Figure 4**).[1] This predisposition is related to the eccentric scaphoid ossification that begins within the distal pole and propagates toward the proximal pole, thus rendering the distal third more susceptible to fracture.[57]

The predominance of distal third scaphoid fractures has been verified by numerous studies. D'Arienzo[56] reported on 39 scaphoid fractures in children and noted that 31 involved the distal third. Thirty-one fractures were type III, 6 were type II, and only 2 were type I (purely chondral). In a similar study, Mussbichler[2] analyzed scaphoid fractures in 100 children younger than 15 years of age. Fifty-two were avulsion fractures of the dorsoradial aspect of the distal end, 33 were fractures through the distal third, and only 15 were fractures

about the waist. In another study, Vahvanen and Westerlund[1] analyzed 108 pediatric scaphoid fractures and found 49% involved the distal third of the bone, with 38% of those avulsion fractures.

FIGURE 5

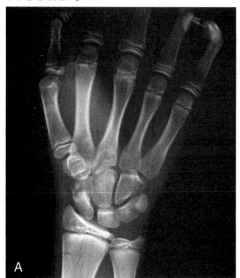 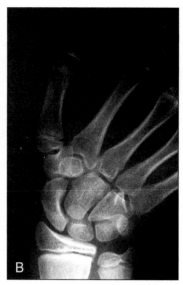 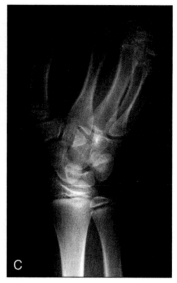

A, PA radiograph of the right wrist in a 12-year-old boy who fell while playing ice hockey and reported pain in that wrist and shoulder reveals a distal pole scaphoid fracture with slight comminution. Radiographs of shoulder revealed a distal third clavicle fracture. Scaphoid **(B)** and pronated oblique **(C)** views obtained after 8 weeks of casting demonstrate fracture healing. (Courtesy of Shriners Hospital for Children, Philadelphia, PA.)

TREATMENT

Acute Fracture

Most pediatric scaphoid fractures can be treated with cast immobilization because children's bones possess a great ability to heal and remodel. In addition, most scaphoid fractures in children are either incomplete (disrupting only a single cortex) or nondisplaced. This principle is especially true for the distal pole, which is the most common site of scaphoid fracture (**Figure 5, A**).[1,2,5,10,40] Therefore, cast immobilization is the gold standard of treatment for most nondisplaced or minimally displaced pediatric scaphoid fractures (**Figure 5, B and C**).[58-60] For avulsion and incomplete fractures, a short thumb spica cast for 4 to 6 weeks is recommended. In the young child, a long arm cast is appropriate to prevent the cast from sliding off the arm. For complete distal third and waist fractures, 6 to 8 weeks of immobilization is recommended.

A longer period of immobilization (8 to 12 weeks) is recommended for proximal pole fractures, delayed diagnosis, or fractures with apparent bony resorption (**Figure 6**).[44] Immobilization usually begins with 6 weeks in

FIGURE 6

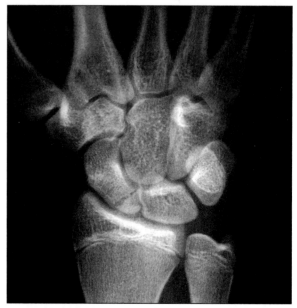

PA radiograph of a 16-year-old male hockey player with a proximal third scaphoid fracture. (Courtesy of Shriners Hospital for Children, Philadelphia, PA.)

FIGURE 7

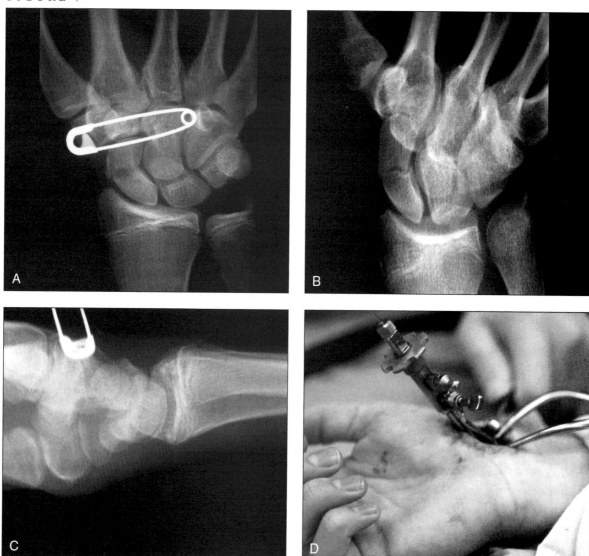

PA **(A)**, scaphoid **(B)**, and lateral **(C)** radiographs of a 13-year-old hockey player with persistent pain after diagnosis of a wrist sprain show a displaced scaphoid nonunion affecting the waist. **D**, A volar approach for bone grafting and screw fixation was used. (Courtesy of Shriners Hospital for Children, Philadelphia, PA.)

a long thumb spica cast, followed by 6 weeks of a short thumb spica cast.[1,41]

Nonunion

The distal and retrograde blood supply of the scaphoid does not change with growth.[60] Because most pediatric scaphoid fractures involve the distal third fractures, frac-

ture union is predictable and nonunion is uncommon.[62-69] The risk of nonunion and osteonecrosis is higher with more proximal fractures. Factors contributing to nonunion are delayed presentation and/or failure of initial diagnosis coupled with continued motion across the fracture site. Most reported pediatric scaphoid nonunions involve the waist (**Figure 7**).[67-69] Pediatric scaphoid nonunion can be managed in multiple ways.

FIGURE 7 (CONT)

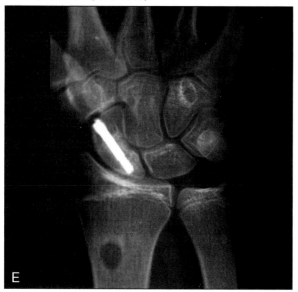 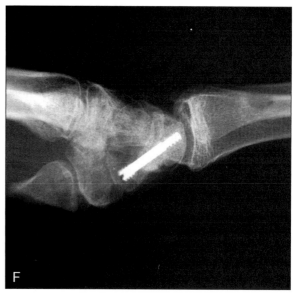

Postoperative PA **(E)** and lateral **(F)** radiographs after bone grafting and screw fixation show bony consolidation. (Courtesy of Shriners Hospital for Children, Philadelphia, PA.)

Union has been achieved by casting alone,[70] casting with pulse electromagnetic field,[64] Matti-Russe procedure,[68,71] open reduction with bone grafting alone,[69] bone grafting, and Kirschner wire fixation,[58] and open reduction using a compression screw with or without bone grafting.[67]

Horii and associates[72] reported a large series of scaphoid fractures (64 patients) that included 46 instances of nonunion. The mechanisms of injury primarily were sporting activities, fighting, and punching game machines. All nonunions were waist fractures, except for one proximal and one distal pole fracture. The patients were between 11 and 15 years of age and often presented late. There were numerous reasons for delayed presentation, including a reluctance to tell their parents about their mechanism of injury, moderate symptoms that were not severe enough to seek medical attention, and a fear of losing a position on a sporting team.

Fabre and colleagues[73] reviewed fractures and nonunions of the carpal scaphoid in children. They evaluated the literature and noted a low nonunion rate (0.8%) for acute scaphoid fractures treated with immobilization.[74,75] Their own series of 23 acute fractures all healed with cast immobilization with instances of scaphoid nonunion only in patients referred from other institutions who presented late (mean, 7 to 11 months). Both patients were treated successfully with cast immobilization. Wilson-MacDonald[16] also recommended a trial of cast immobilization as the initial treatment in cases of delayed or nonunion.

Mintzer and Waters[76] reported a series of 13 scaphoid nonunions in children (ages 9 to 15 years), and all involved the scaphoid waist. The mechanism of injury was a fall on the outstretched arm in all patients; 9 of the 13 fractures occurred during a sporting event. Preferred treatment was surgical intervention. The average time between fracture and surgery was 16.7 months. All nonunions united after surgical stabilization, with an average follow-up of 6.9 years. Four nonunions were treated using the Matti-Russe procedure, and nine were treated with Herbert screw fixation combined with iliac crest bone grafting. All cases resulted in clinical and radiographic union with range of motion and strength similar to the contralateral wrist. In cases of unclear union, CT can be used to assess trabeculae crossing the fracture site (**Figure 8**).

Toh and associates[24] reported their experience man-

FIGURE 8

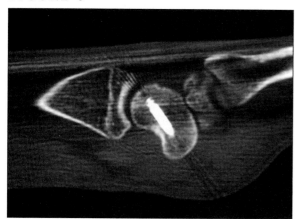

Postoperative CT scan confirms crossing trabeculae across the fracture site. (Courtesy of Shriners Hospital for Children, Philadelphia, PA.)

aging 64 pediatric scaphoid fractures. Forty-six were fracture nonunions. Patient age ranged from 11 to 15 years, and the average duration from injury to surgery was 74 days (range, 42 to 210 days). The average time of follow-up was 27 months. Surgical indications included acute unstable fractures, fibrous union, and established pseudarthrosis. Surgery consisted of cannulated screw fixation in 52 cases, including 35 cases of bone graft. All but two cases achieved solid bony union. The functional outcomes were not statistically significantly different between the acute cohort and the nonacute group. In the two patients with persistent nonunion, one patient was an ice hockey player who was noncompliant with immobilization. He required a secondary bone grafting to achieve bony union. In the other patient, a persistent nonunion developed that necessitated repeat Herbert screw fixation and bone grafting to achieve bony union.

Complications

No major complications have been reported from surgical intervention of scaphoid fractures in children. However, concern has been raised regarding the possibility of disturbing the normal growth of the scaphoid with screw fixation.[24] Previous reports have suggested that smaller scaphoid screws may be preferred to accommodate the pediatric scaphoid and still provide rigid internal fixation.[76] In all reported pediatric patients

treated with screw fixation, patient age was 11 years or older. There is no report that explores the youngest age that allows safe screw fixation.

Osteonecrosis of the proximal part of the scaphoid is possible, but rare in children.[7] This is attributed to the dominance of distal pole fractures and that restoration of blood supply may occur more readily in the child.

Scaphoid malunion resulting in humpback deformity is a known complication among adult patients with a displaced scaphoid fracture. Subsequently, the lunate extends and a dorsal intercalated segmental instability results with limited wrist range of motion.[77] Correction of this deformity in adults involves osteotomy and bone grafting to restore the normal configuration of the scaphoid.[78] Because a child's bone has great ability to remodel, healing of a scaphoid malunion and correction of an intercalated instability pattern often are possible without the need for corrective osteotomy.[78]

CONCLUSIONS

Scaphoid fractures in children are uncommon. A high index of suspicion is required when clinical signs and symptoms support a scaphoid fracture in a child. Initially, radiographic evaluation with multiple views is necessary to assess for fracture. If necessary, advanced imaging studies, such as MRI, should be obtained. Most pediatric scaphoid fractures can be treated with cast immobilization, which typically results in healing. Scaphoid nonunion usually is the result of delayed presentation or missed diagnosis. Fortunately, union can be reliably achieved with recognition and appropriate treatment.

REFERENCES

1. Vahvanen V, Westerlund M: Fracture of the carpal scaphoid in children: A clinical and roentgenological study of 108 cases. *Acta Orthop Scand* 1980;51:909-913.

2. Mussbichler H: Injuries of the carpal scaphoid in children. *Acta Radiol* 1961;56:110-115.

3. Nafie SA: Fractures of the carpal bones in children. *Injury* 1987;18:117-119.

4. Kocher MS, Waters PM, Micheli LJ: Upper extremity injuries in the pediatric athlete. *Sports Med* 2000;30:117-135.

5. Christodoulou AG, Colton CL: Scaphoid fractures in children. *J Pediatric Orthop* 1986;6:37-39.

6. Greene MH, Hadied AM, LaMont RL: Scaphoid fractures in children. *J Hand Surg Am* 1984;9:536-541.

7. Larson B, Light TR, Ogden JA: Fracture and ischemic necrosis of the immature scaphoid. *J Hand Surg* 1987;12:122-127.

8. Light TR: Injury to the immature carpus. *Hand Clin* 1988;4:415-424.

9. Mazet R, Hohl M: Fractures of the carpal navicular: Analysis of ninety-one cases and review of the literature. *J Bone Joint Surg Am* 1963;45:82-112.

10. Wulff R, Schmidt T: Carpal fractures in children. *J Pediatr Orthop* 1998;18:462-465.

11. Bloem JJ: Fractures of the carpal scaphoid in a child aged 4. *Arch Chir Neerlandicum* 1971;23:92-94.

12. Light TR: Carpal injuries in children. *Hand Clin* 2000;16:513-522.

13. Gamble JG, Simmons SC: Bilateral scaphoid fractures in a child. *Clin Orthop* 1982;162:125-128.

14. D'Arienzo M: Scaphoid fractures in children. *J Hand Surg Br* 2002;27:5:424-426.

15. Cockshott WP: Distal avulsion fractures of the scaphoid. *Br J Radiol* 1980;53:1037-1040.

16. Wilson-Macdonald J: Delayed union of the distal scaphoid in children. *J Hand Surg Am* 1987;12:520-522.

17. Stanciu C, Dumont A: Changing patterns of scaphoid fractures in adolescents. *Can J Surg* 1994;37:214-216.

18. Stuart HC, Pyle SI, Cornoni J, Reed RB: Onsets, completions and spans of ossification in the 20 bone growth centers of the hand and wrist. *Pediatrics* 1962;29:237-249.

19. Gruber W: Os naviculare carpi bipartitum. *Arch Pathol Anat* 1877;69:391-396.

20. Pfitzner W: Beiträge zur Kenntniss des menschlichen Extremitatenskelets. VI. Die Variationen im Aufbau des Handskelets. *Morph Arb* 1895;4:347-570.

21. Pfitzner, W. (1900) Die morphologischen Elemente des menschlichen Handskeletts. *Ztschr f Morphol Anthropol* 1900;2:77, 365.

22. Louis DS, Calhoun TP, Garn SM, Carroll RE, Burdi AR: Congenital bipartite scaphoid: Fact or fiction? *J Bone Joint Surg Am* 1976;58:1108-1111.

23. Goddard N: Carpal fractures in children. *Clin Orthop* 2005;432:73-76.

24. Toh S, Miura H, Arai K, Yasumura M, Wada M: Scaphoid fractures in children: Problems and treatment. *J Pediatr Orthop* 2003;23:216-221.

25. Takka S, Poyraz A: Enchondroma of the scaphoid bone. *Arch Orthop Trauma Surg* 2002;122:369-370.

26. Malizos KN, Getalis ID, Ioachim EE, Soucacos PN: Pathologic fracture of the scaphoid due to enchondroma: Treatment with vascularized bone grafting. Report of a case. *J Hand Surg Am* 1998;23:334-337.

27. Masada K, Fujiwara K, Yoshikawa H, Iwaki K: Chondroma of the scaphoid. *J Bone Joint Surg Br* 1989;71:705-708.

28. Minkowitz B, Patel M, Minkowitz S: Scaphoid enchondroma. *Orthop Rev* 1992;21:1241-1244.

29. Redfem DRM, Forester AJ, Evans MS, Sohail M: Enchondroma of the scaphoid. *J Hand Surg Br* 1997;22:235-236.

30. Takigawa K: Chondromas of the bones of the hand: A review of 110 cases. *J Bone Joint Surg Am* 1971;53:1591-1600.

31. Sawant M, Miller J: Scaphocapitate syndrome in an adolescent. *J Hand Surg Am* 2000;25:1096-1099.

32. Fenton RL: The naviculo-capitate fracture syndrome. *J Bone Joint Surg Am* 1956;38:681-684.

33. Anderson WJ: Simultaneous fracture of the scaphoid and capitate in a child. *J Hand Surg Am* 1987;12:271-273.

34. Milliez PY, Dallaserra M, Thomine JM: An unusual variety of scapho-capitate syndrome. *J Hand Surg Br* 1993;18:53-57.

35. Compson JP: Trans-carpal injuries associated with distal radial fractures in children: A series of three cases. *J Hand Surg Br* 1992;17:311-314.

36. Hokan R, Bryce GM, Cobb NJ: Dislocation of scaphoid and fractured capitate in a child. *Injury* 1993;24:496-497.

37. Kamano M, Fukushima K, Honda Y: Multiple carpal bone fractures in an eleven-year-old. *J Orthop Trauma* 1998;12:445-448.

38. Nashi M, Manjunath B, Banerjee RD, Creedon RJ: Supracondylar fracture of the humerus with ipsilateral fracture of the scaphoid in a child. *J Accid Emerg Med* 1998;15:431.

39. Stanitski CL, Micheli LS: Simultaneous ipsilateral fractures of the arm and forearm in children. *Clin Orthop* 1980;153:218-221.

40. Greene WB, Anderson WJ: Simultaneous fracture of the scaphoid and radius in a child. *J Pediatr Orthop* 1982;2:191-194.

41. Sherwin JM, Nagel DA, Southwick WO: Bipartite carpal navicular and the diagnostic problem of bone partition: A case report. *J Trauma* 1967;11:440-443.

42. Albert MC, Barre PS: A scaphoid fracture associated with a displaced distal radial fracture in child. *Clin Orthop* 1989;240:232-235.

43. DeCoster TA, Faherty S, Morris AL: Pediatric carpal fracture dislocation: Case report. *J Orthop Trauma* 1994;8:76-78.

44. Pick RY, Segal D: Carpal scaphoid fracture and nonunion in an eight-year-old child. *J Bone Joint Surg Am* 1982;12:441-443.

45. Chen SC: The scaphoid compression test. *J Hand Surg Br* 1989;4:323-325.

46. Bohler E, Trojan E, Jahna H: The results of treatment of 734 fresh, simple fractures of the scaphoid. *J Hand Surg Br* 2003;28:219:331.

47. Leicht P, Mikkelsen JB, Larsen CF: Scapholunate distance in children. *Acta Radiol* 1996;37:625-626.

48. Swezey RL, Alexander SJ: Notching of the carpal navicular. *Ann Rheum Dis* 1969;28:45-48.

49. Cook PA, Kobus RJ, Wiand W: Scapholunate ligament disruption in a skeletally immature patient: A case report. *J Hand Surg Am* 1997;22:83-85.

50. Cook PA, Yu JS, Wiand W: Suspected scaphoid fractures in skeletally immature patients: Application of MRI. *J Comput Assist Tomogr* 1997;21:511-515.

51. Johnson KJ, Haigh SF, Symonds KE: MRI in the management of scaphoid fractures in skeletally immature patients. *Pediatr Radiol* 2000;30:685-688.

52. Waizenegger M, Wastie ML, Barton NJ, Davis TR: Scintigraphy in the evaluation of the "clinical" scaphoid fracture. *J Hand Surg Br* 1994;19:750-753.

53. Bain GI, Bennett JD, Richards RS, Slethaugh GP, Roth JH: Longitudinal computed tomography of the scaphoid: A new technique. *Skeletal Radiol* 1995;24:271-273.

54. Dias JJ, Hui ACW, Lamont AC: Real time ultrasonography in the assessment of movement at the site of a scaphoid fracture non-union. *J Hand Surg Br* 1994;19:498-504.

55. Senall JA, Failla JM, Bouffard A, Holsbeeck MV: Ultrasound for the early diagnosis of clinically suspected scaphoid fracture. *J Hand Surg Am* 2004;29:400-405.

56. D'Arienzo M: Scaphoid fractures in children. *J Hand Surg Br* 2002;27:424-426.

57. Grundy M: Fractures of the carpal scaphoid in children. A series of eight cases. *Br J Surg* 1969;56:523-524.

58. Maxted MJ, Owen R: Two cases of non-union of carpal scaphoid fractures in children. *Injury* 1982;12:441-443.

59. Ogden JA: *Skeletal Injury in the Child*. Philadelphia, PA, Lea & Febiger, 1982, pp 363-364.

60. Stewart MJ: Fracture of the carpal navicular (scaphoid). *J Bone Joint Surg Am* 1954;36:998-1006.

61. Taleisnik J, Kelly PJ: The extraosseous and intraosseous blood supply of the scaphoid bone. *J Bone Joint Surg Am* 1966;48:1125-1137.

62. Barton NJ: Apparent and partial non-union of the scaphoid. *J Hand Surg Br* 1996;21:496-500.

63. DeCoster TA, Faherty S, Morris AL: Case report: Pediatric carpal dislocation. *J Orthop Trauma* 1994;8:76-78.

64. Godley DR: Nonunited carpal scaphoid fracture in a child: Treatment with pulsed electromagnetic field stimulation. *Orthopedics* 1997;20:718-719.

65. Littlefield WG, Friedman RL, Urbaniak JR: Bilateral non-union of the carpal scaphoid in a child: A case report. *J Bone Joint Surg Am* 1995;77:124-126.

66. Mintzer CM, Waters PM, Simmons BP: Nonunion of the scaphoid in children treated by Herbert screw fixation and bone grafting: A report of five cases. *J Bone Joint Surg Br* 1995;77:98-100.

67. Onuba O, Ireland J: Two cases of nonunion of fractures of the scaphoid in children. *Injury* 1984;15:109-112.

68. Southcott R, Rosman MA: Nonunion of carpal scaphoid fractures in children. *J Bone Joint Surg Br* 1977;59:20-23.

69. Caputo AE, Watson HK, Nissen C: Scaphoid nonunion in a child: A case report. *J Hand Surg Am* 1995;20:243-245.

70. De Boeck H, Van Wellen P, Haentjens P: Nonunion of a carpal scaphoid fracture in a child. *J Orthop Trauma* 1991;5:370-372.

71. Russe O: Fracture of the carpal navicular: Diagnosis, nonoperative, and operative treatment. *J Bone Joint Surg Am* 1960;42:759-768.

72. Horii E, Nakamura R, Watanabe K: Scaphoid fracture as a "puncher's fracture." *J Orthop Trauma* 1994;8:107-110.

73. Fabre O, De Boek H, Haentjens P: Fractures and nonunions of the carpal scaphoid in children. *Acta Orthop Belg* 2001;67:121-125.

74. Langhoff O, Andersen JL: Consequences of late immobilization of scaphoid fractures. *J Bone Joint Surg Br* 1988;13:77-79.

75. Stanciu C, Dumont A: Changing patterns of scaphoid fractures in adolescents. *Can J Surg* 1994;37:214-216.

76. Mintzer CM, Waters PM: Surgical treatment of pediatric scaphoid fracture nonunions. *J Pediatr Orthop* 1999;19:236-239.

77. Nakamura R, Imaeda T, Miura T: Scaphoid malunion. *J Bone Joint Surg Br* 1991;73:124-137.

78. Amadio PC, Berquist TH, Smith DK, Ilstrup DM, Cooney WP, Linscheid RL: Scaphoid malunion. *J Hand Surg Am* 1989;14:679-687.

79. Suzuki K, Herbert TJ: Spontaneous correction of dorsal intercalated segment instability deformity with scaphoid malunion in the skeletally immature. *J Hand Surg Am* 1993;18:1012-1015.

CHAPTER 8

LONG-STANDING SCAPHOID NONUNIONS

STEVEN L. MORAN, MD

Nonunion of the scaphoid may occur after a delay in diagnosis, inadequate fixation, osteonecrosis, or biomechanical stresses across the fracture site. Nonunions may remain asymptomatic or minimally symptomatic for long periods of time with the patient presenting years after the initiating trauma. In such cases, the chances of primary scaphoid repair may be poor; in addition, biomechanical alterations within the carpus may result in osteoarthritis.

When a patient presents with wrist arthritis after a scaphoid nonunion, obtaining scaphoid union alone does not provide adequate pain relief postoperatively. In many cases, the scaphoid is beyond repair. In such cases, wrist salvage procedures are necessary to preserve the remaining radiocarpal motion, reduce pain, and return the patient to a more functional status. This chapter reviews the pathophysiology of scaphoid nonunion arthritis and provides an overview of treatment options.

PATHOPHYSIOLOGY OF CARPAL ARTHRITIS AFTER SCAPHOID NONUNION

The scaphoid bridges both the proximal and distal carpal rows. As such it is subject to opposing forces at both its distal and proximal poles. With long-standing midwaist or proximal pole fractures, the scaphoid tends to collapse under the strain of these opposing forces. The distal portion of the scaphoid assumes a flexed posture under the load of the thumb axis and distal carpal row, and the

proximal component, still attached to the lunate (through a presumably intact scapholunate interosseous ligament) tends to extend through the pull of the lunate and triquetrum. The humpback deformity that develops in cases of scaphoid malunion is the result of scaphoid healing within this collapsed posture[1-3] (Figure 1).

Smith and colleagues[4,5] simulated unstable scaphoid fractures in five cadaveric wrists. The scaphoid tended to assume a humpback pattern in all wrist positions after osteotomy; however, the greatest angulation occurred with wrist flexion. Viegas and colleagues[6] simulated proximal pole osteotomies to examine load distribution changes across the carpus. Their results showed no significant increase in load at the radiolunate joint or below the proximal pole articulation; however, there was an increase in contact pressure and overall contact area between the distal scaphoid fragment and the radius.[6] This correlates directly with the first and second radiographic stages of scaphoid nonunion arthritis, which develop at the styloid and at the distal radioscaphoid fossa.

The proximal portion of the fractured scaphoid often is unable to balance the extension forces transmitted to the lunate by the triquetrum; this results in an extended posture of the lunate with concomitant capitate flexion or dorsal intercalated segment instability (DISI) as seen on lateral radiographs[2,7] (Figure 2). Carpal instability and DISI posturing predispose to the development of midcarpal arthritis. The incidence of carpal instability associated with scaphoid nonunion has been reported at 22% to 68%.[8-10] Moritomo and colleagues,[11] with the

FIGURE 1

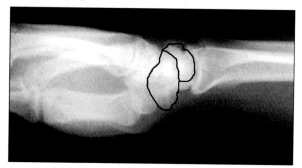

Lateral radiograph shows a humpback deformity of the scaphoid (outline) resulting from an untreated scaphoid fracture.

FIGURE 2

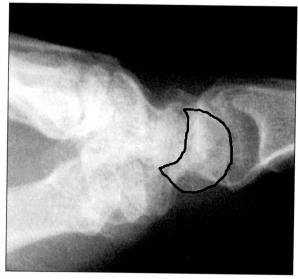

DISI posture of the lunate (outline) in a 9-month-old scaphoid nonunion.

aid of three-dimensional CT, examined scaphoid fracture patterns to determine whether fracture location contributed to the development of carpal instability. These authors concluded that fracture location proximal or distal to the scaphoid's dorsal ridge influenced the development of carpal instability. The dorsal intercarpal (DIC) ligament attaches at the scaphoid's dorsal ridge. Fractures distal to the DIC ligament insertion were thought to flex under the load of the trapezium, whereas fractures that occurred proximal to the dorsal ridge preserved the ligamentous attachments of the DIC ligament to the distal pole. The preserved ligament helps to maintain the distal fragment in an extended position, leading to a lower incidence of DISI deformity.[11]

IMAGING AND CLASSIFICATION

The radiographic progression of radiocarpal arthritis in long-standing scaphoid nonunions is similar to the arthritis pattern seen in the scapholunate advanced collapse (SLAC) wrist, originally described by Watson.[12,13] Scaphoid nonunion arthritis is described in a three-stage progression. Stage I is characterized by arthritic changes and osteophyte formation at the radial styloid, consistent with the biomechanical findings of Viegas and associates.[6] In stage II, arthritis develops at the radioscaphoid joint. In stage III, patients have arthritic involvement of the capitolunate joint. This progression has been termed scaphoid nonunion advanced collapse (SNAC wrist).[10,13,14] The articular surface beneath the proximal pole of the lunate tends to remain free of arthritic changes as it moves in conjunction with the lunate through an intact scapholunate interosseous ligament (Figure 3).

TREATMENT

Historically, it was thought that the asymptomatic patient with an established nonunion and no carpal collapse[15] did not require treatment.[16-20] However, a growing number of publications have reported that, over time, ununited fractures increase the risk for osteoarthritis and impaired wrist motion.[8-10,21-25] In counseling my patients with relatively asymptomatic scaphoid nonunions, I presume that few nonunions will remain stable, nondisplaced, or free of arthritis after 10 years; however, studies on the natural history of scaphoid nonunion are limited.[26] Nonetheless, with the amount of biomechanical data available, it is logical to assume that the progression to radiocarpal arthritis is more frequent in patients with displaced fractures and coexisting carpal instability.

Scaphoid Preservation Versus Wrist Salvage

Radiocarpal arthritis generally is the principal reason for a wrist salvage procedure. In such cases, attempts at obtaining scaphoid union, even if successful, can result in persistent wrist pain. In patients with long-standing

FIGURE 3

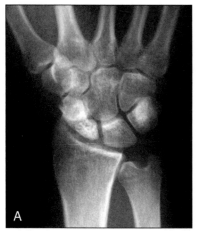 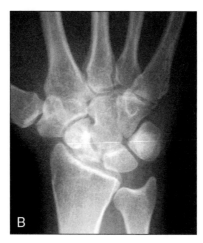 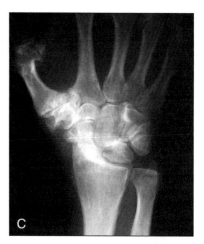

A, PA radiograph shows radioscaphoid arthritis in a patient with stage II SNAC arthritis. Stage III SNAC is defined by the presence of degenerative changes within the midcarpal joint (**B** and **C**).

nonunion in the absence of significant arthritic changes, the choice of scaphoid salvage should be predicated on the duration of the nonunion, scaphoid vascularity, and evidence of carpal instability.

Recently, several authors have discussed prognostic factors for the healing of scaphoid nonunions. A multicenter study by Schuind and associates[27] of 138 patients, reported that heavy laborers, nonunions present for more than 5 years, and a short period of postoperative immobilization lead to an increased risk of persistent nonunion. Patients who require styloidectomy also tend to have a poorer outcome, perhaps resulting from preexisting radiocarpal arthritis or the destabilization of the carpus after large styloidectomy. Shaw and Jones[28] and Inoue and co-workers[29,30] also have found that the longer the nonunion is present, the lower the surgical success rate. Shaw and Jones reported that union rates were 80% if the nonunion was treated within 5 years but decreased to 50% if the nonunion had been present for more than 5 years. Additional factors associated with lower healing rates included the presence of osteonecrosis and previous scaphoid surgery.

The vascular status of the proximal fragment has a major impact on nonunion outcome; however, it is difficult to evaluate proximal pole vascularity preoperatively.[31-33] Increased radiographic density of the proximal pole correlates poorly with proximal pole blood flow when correlated with MRI.[34-36] Even standard MRI is not reliable for consistently predicting which proximal pole fracture will heal.[37] A better assessment of proximal pole vascularity is provided with dynamic gadolinium-enhanced MRI, which has 83% accuracy when compared to actual intraoperative punctate bleeding.[38] In cases of significant avascularity, vascularized bone grafting or conventional wedge grafting may be attempted.

Wrist Salvage and Palliative Procedures

Salvage procedures are necessary when bone grafting fails or arthritis has developed within the wrist joint. In such cases, there are multiple options for wrist salvage and should be guided by the stage of SNAC arthritis, patient occupation, and tolerance for surgery.

Radial Styloidectomy

For patients with early SNAC wrist, where arthritis is confined to the radial styloid, radial styloidectomy may be combined with attempts at scaphoid salvage. Radial styloidectomy is usually performed subperiosteally through the anatomic snuffbox but also may be performed arthroscopically as a palliative procedure. Care must be taken to preserve the important volar radial ligament attachments; if more than 6 to 10 mm of styloid is removed, the radioscaphocapitate ligament origin

FIGURE 4

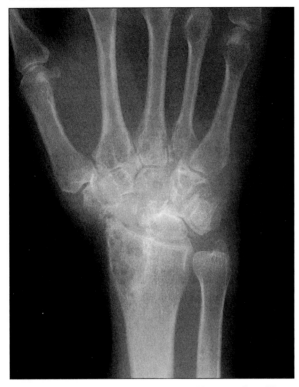

Silicone synovitis developed in this wrist 10 years after silicone scaphoid replacement. Note the presence of bone cyst throughout the radial styloid and degenerative changes throughout the midcarpal joint.

becomes significantly compromised, possibly resulting in ulnar translation of the carpus.[39,40] The radial styloid fragment may be used as a bone graft.[41,42] Styloidectomy alone has been unsatisfactory[19,43] but is successful when combined with bone grafts, with or without internal fixation for scaphoid salvage.[19,41,43-45]

Scaphoid Replacement and Silicone Particle Synovitis
Silicone prosthesis has been recommended for the treatment recalcitrant nonunions and proximal pole fractures. Results have been tempered by the development of silicone synovitis. The problem is increasingly being reported as longer term follow-up of silicone implants of carpal bones and wrists is available, even causing some early proponents of silicone implant arthroplasty to reverse their support of the procedure.[46-48]

Silicone synovitis describes the inflammatory arthropathy seen in some patients after silicone implant arthroplasty, particularly of the wrist or carpal bones.[49-55] The pathophysiology appears to relate to microparticulate fragmentation of the implant. All silicone polymers fragment when abraded; this is a particular risk in load-bearing implants such as those of the wrist. Clinically, the manifestations are those of an inflammatory synovitis around the implant; radiographically, osteopenia and later cyst formation are noted. On surgical exploration, proliferative synovitis invading bone is often seen. Histologically, the synovitis is characterized by macrophages containing engulfed silicone particles.

Despite these concerns, recent long-term follow-up reports have suggested that a percentage of patients remains asymptomatic despite ongoing carpal arthrosis and progressive silicone synovitis. Haussman[46] reported on 11 patients with follow-up of up to 16 years. Two patients required implant removal. The remaining nine all showed radiographic evidence of silicone synovitis and advancing arthrosis; however, the majority had minimal symptoms. Vinnars and colleagues[56] examined 32 patients undergoing silicone implant arthroplasty between 1974 and 1988. In their study, 25% of patients underwent removal for implant failure at 10 years. More than 50% of the remaining patients showed evidence of interosseous cyst formation on final follow-up. Nine of the 21 patients reported little to no pain.[56] All patients with silicone implants in place should be advised of the possibility of silicone synovitis. For patients with implants in place without evidence of silicone synovitis, regular follow-up, either annually or biannually, is advised (**Figure 4**).

Neurectomy
For those patients in whom major surgery is contraindicated or those patients who refuse partial or total wrist fusion, selective wrist neurectomy may offer some improvement in wrist pain. Selective neurectomy of the anterior and posterior interosseous nerves has been shown to provide partial relief of wrist pain in patients with radiocarpal arthritis.[57] More definitive attempts at wrist denervation may also be attempted; however, total pain relief is difficult to achieve.[58] We have found that preoperative marcaine block of the anterior and posterior interosseous nerves provides the patient with a reasonable assessment of postoperative pain relief.

FIGURE 5

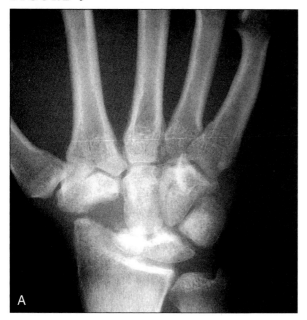
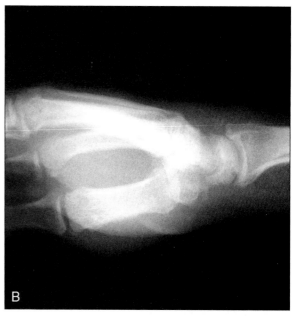

PA **(A)** and lateral **(B)** radiographs of a 52-year-old contractor who refused four-corner fusion but underwent distal scaphoid resection. Note evidence of mild dorsiflexion of the lunate in the lateral view.

Bentzon's Procedure

This operation was initially used by Bentzon in 1939 and was first reported in 1944.[59] The concept is to convert a painful nonunion into a pain-free pseudarthrosis by placing a soft-tissue flap based on the dorsoradial aspect of the wrist between the fragments. Although Bentzon's procedure has failed to become popular outside of Scandinavia,[60,61] results appear comparable to those obtained after bone grafting.[62] A long-term review showed good results 22 to 39 years after Bentzon's operation.[63] Carpal collapse, found in 15 of 26 patients, and osteoarthritis, present in 7, did not result in clinical disability. This procedure may still be considered a satisfactory alternative when prolonged immobilization is contraindicated and after bone graft procedures have failed.

Distal Scaphoid Resection

Excision of the distal scaphoid has been recommended for degenerative arthritis and pain in long-standing nonunions.[64,65] The benefits of distal scaphoid resection are its technical ease and short period of immobilization. This procedure may be performed through a volar, lateral, or arthroscopic approach.[66] The procedure does not preclude proximal row carpectomy (PRC) or four-corner fusion if it is unsuccessful.

Malerich and associates[64] noted an 85% improvement in wrist motion and a 134% increase in grip strength over a 49-month follow-up period. This procedure generally is not appropriate for patients with ongoing capitolunate arthritis, significant wrist instability, or DISI deformity; however, Soejima and colleagues[67] recently reported their 2-year results with this procedure in nine patients who had evidence of preexisting radioscaphoid or capitolunate arthritis. All patients had good to excellent results based on the modified Mayo wrist scoring system. Four patients had no pain, and the remaining five had only mild pain with strenuous activities. Significant midcarpal arthritis developed in one patient. Long-term progression to midcarpal arthritis has yet to be determined, but at present the short-term data for this procedure are comparable with, if not superior to, many other salvage options (**Figure 5**).

Proximal Row Carpectomy

In PRC, the intercalary proximal carpal row is removed, turning the wrist into a simple hinge joint. The capitate is allowed to articulate within the lunate facet of the radius. The radius of curvature of the capitate is larger than that of the lunate; thus, there is incongruity at the new articulation, which predisposes to articular wear. Ideally, the lunate facet of the radius and capitate should be free of arthritic changes for best results. This procedure is not indicated in advanced SNAC wrist where midcarpal arthritis is present. In such cases, intercarpal fusion is recommended.

Hill[68] reported that PRC was indicated in older patients with symptomatic scaphoid nonunions who did not wish to accept a long period of immobilization; others have used this treatment for younger, active, heavy laborers with very good functional and clinical results.[69-72] Krakauer and associates[14] compared proximal row carpectomy with intercarpal fusion and found that carpectomy preserved motion better, an average arc of 71° versus 54° for limited arthrodesis. Both procedures preserved reasonable strength and reduced pain.

Studies examining the long-term outcomes of this procedure specifically for scaphoid nonunion are limited. Jebson and colleagues[73] reported on 20 patients, 11 of whom underwent PRC for scaphoid nonunion. Two patients in this series required wrist arthrodesis for persistent pain. The remaining 18 patients were evaluated at an average of 13 years after surgery. The average wrist range of motion and the average maximal grip strength were 63% and 83%, respectively, of the opposite extremity. Of the 18 patients, 16 had returned to their previous employment. Flattening of the capitate was present in 33% of patients. In addition, 22% of patients had some evidence of moderate to severe radiocapitate arthrosis; however, this did not correlate with patient satisfaction or wrist pain.

DiDonna and colleagues[74] also examined 10-year follow-up for PRC. In their study, 22 wrists were followed for an average of 14 years. Six wrists had the original diagnosis of SNAC arthritis. There were four failures (18%) requiring fusion at an average of 7 years after the initial surgery; two occurred in patients with SNAC wrists. The average flexion extension arc was 72°, with an average grip strength of 91% of the contralateral side. Of the 18 wrists that did not fail, all patients were either satisfied or very satisfied with the procedure, with an overall Disabilities of the Arm, Shoulder, and Hand (DASH) score of 9. Degenerative changes were seen in

14 of 17 wrists at follow-up, but this did not correlate with symptoms.

Partial Arthrodesis (Four-Corner and Other)

Both Sutro[75] and Helfet[76] proposed to treat scaphoid nonunions by arthrodesing both fragments to the capitate when there is extensive sclerosis or resorption of the fragments or degenerative changes between the scaphoid and capitate. When the radiocarpal joint shows signs of osteoarthritis but the scaphocapitate joint is satisfactory, radioscapholunate fusion may be considered instead.[778] Other types of limited arthrodesis have been proposed.[78] I believe that most scaphoid nonunions can be satisfactorily treated with techniques other than limited arthrodesis. However, these may be indicated as salvage procedures, particularly after repeated failures of bone grafts and to prevent midcarpal collapse in unstable wrists when scaphoid excision is considered. For the common combination of radioscaphoid and midcarpal arthritis often seen in chronic nonunions or significant malunions, a combination of midcarpal arthrodesis and scaphoid excision can be considered.[12,79] Although this SNAC wrist procedure was initially proposed to be used with a silicone scaphoid implant, scaphoid excision without an implant works equally well.[80-82] Watson and Ballet[12] and later Watson and Ryu[83] stated that the proposed advantages of four-corner fusion over PRC are retention of the radiolunate interface and preservation of carpal height, which presumably maintains the resting muscle tension across the wrist-preserving grip strength.

Several studies have examined the functional outcome after four-corner fusion.[14,84-87] Ashmead and associates[84] provided one of the largest series, reporting on 100 cases. In their series, final wrist flexion-extension arc averaged 53% of the contralateral side and final grip strength averaged 80% of the contralateral side. Nonunion occurred in only 3% of patients; 51% of patients had total resolution of wrist pain, whereas 15% continued to have pain with daily activities or at rest.

Techniques ensuring successful outcome have focused on adequate decortication of the four bony surfaces and correction of the dorsiflexed lunate to reestablish a collinear relationship between the lunate and capitate. Failure to correct lunate position can lead to limited wrist extension, hardware abutment, and pain (**Figure 6**).[84,85] The use of bone graft has not been shown to clearly correlate with fusion rates nor has hardware

FIGURE 6

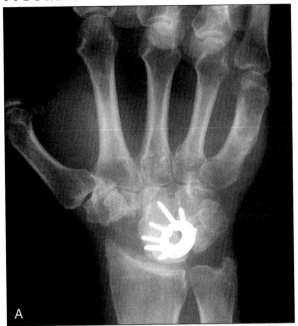

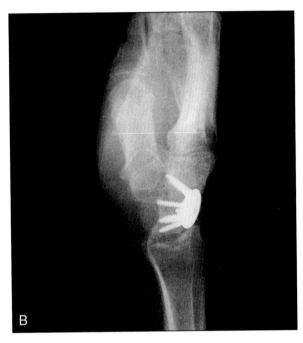

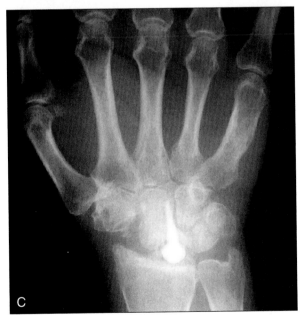

PA **(A)** and lateral **(B)** radiographs of a 58-year-old patient who was referred for persistent wrist pain despite four-corner fusion show nonunion at the fusion mass, persistent DISI positioning of the lunate, and evidence of radiolunate arthritis. **C,** The patient refused total wrist fusion, opting for salvage with a pyrocarbon metacarpal phalangeal implant fitted to replace the degenerative head of the lunate.

choice (D Dennison, AY Shin, SL Moran, et al, presented at the American Academy of Orthopaedic Surgeons annual meeting, Chicago, Illinois, 2006); however, hardware complications have been noted with pins, staples, and circular plates.[14,86,87] Vance and associates[88] reported that nonunion and impingement occurred in 48% of patients treated with circular plate fixation compared with a 6% rate with traditional fixation. In addition, plate fixation was associated with a higher rate of patient dissatisfaction.

A variation of four-corner fusion can involve capitolunate arthrodesis alone. Early attempts using this limited arthrodesis were associated with high rates of nonunion, most likely to the result of a smaller fusion mass.[89-91] Calandruccio and colleagues[92] significantly improved upon these results when they combined capitolunate fusion with scaphoid and triquetral excision. The latter may provide for more wrist motion than four-corner fusion, but long-term data are pending.

The Best Choice: PRC or Four-Corner Fusion

The ideal SNAC salvage procedure has yet to be established; however, the two most popular treatment methods remain PRC and scaphoidectomy with four-corner fusion. Wyrick and associates[86] compared 17 patients undergoing four-corner fusion with 11 patients undergoing PRC with 2-year follow-up. Patients undergoing PRC retained 94% of grip strength compared with 74% in the four-corner group. The total arc of motion was 115° in the PRC group and 95° in the four-corner group. The procedure failed in three patients in the four-corner group and two were awaiting fusion. The authors concluded that PRC was the motion-preserving procedure of choice except in patients with advanced midcarpal arthritis.

In contrast to Wyrick and associates' findings, Tomaino and co-workers[85] and Krakauer and associates[14] reported an approximate failure rate of 20% after PRC and a failure rate of less than 10% after four-corner fusion. Imbriglia and associates[93] noted that grip strength equaled or exceeded preoperative grip strength with both procedures. A recent dual cohort study by Cohen and Kozin[87] compared the two procedures and found range of motion to be approximately 80° in both groups with grip strengths of 71% and 79% in the PRC and four-corner groups, respectively. No significant differences were noted between groups for final range of motion, grip strength, and patient satisfaction.

In summary, both procedures provide good pain relief, which results in improved postoperative grip strength, but these procedures failed to restore normal wrist motion. Most agree that PRC is technically easier, requiring no hardware placement and less postoperative immobilization; however, long-term outcome studies evaluating PRC have consistently reported the development of degenerative arthritis between the capitate and radius at 10 years.

Special Considerations in Stage III and Pancarpal Arthritis

In stage III SNAC, midcarpal arthritis precludes the use of PRC, and four-corner fusion is recommended. Salomon and Eaton,[94] however, described a variation of the PRC that can be attempted in patients with midcarpal arthritis. The procedure involves resection of the proximal capitate to produce a more uniform midcarpal joint; this theoretically allows for an even distribution of the radiocarpal forces over the entire distal carpal row. A dorsal capsular flap is used as an interpositional graft between the capitate and radius. In Salomon and Eaton's study, 3 of 12 patients had scaphoid nonunions. At an average follow-up of 55 months, patients demonstrated an improvement in wrist flexion and grip strength. This procedure may be an alternative to four-corner fusion in cases of midcarpal arthritis.

In advanced arthritis, where long-standing DISI deformity may have resulted in arthritis changes within the lunate fossa, wrist arthrodesis and wrist arthroplasty may be the only options for wrist salvage. The choice of wrist arthroplasty depends on the patient's age, activity level, and status of the contralateral wrist. Direct comparisons between the two techniques have been limited, but patients have been shown to tolerate either procedure. However, I still reserve total wrist arthroplasty for lower demand wrists in older patients.[95,96] Total wrist arthrodesis represents an established means of pain relief and maintains strength in patients with pancarpal arthritis. Options of wrist fusion vary, but I prefer to use a dorsal wrist fusion plate.[27,97]

Preferred Method

For patients presenting with early arthritis, I favor distal scaphoid resection if the patient fulfills the following criteria: lack of midcarpal arthritis and minimal DISI posturing of the lunate. In patients with significant carpal instability but no capitate wear, PRC provides a more rapid return to work and preserves wrist motion. However, in patients younger than 35 years of age, consideration is given to immediate four-corner fusion because of the high incidence of capitoradial arthritis,

FIGURE 7

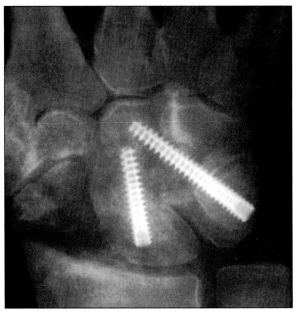

Four-corner fusion performed with two compression screws for the treatment of SNAC.

which appears 8 to 10 years postoperatively.[74]

For younger patients and for those with midcarpal arthritis, a scaphoid excision and four-corner arthrodesis is performed. I prefer to use two compression screws for fusion, although studies have found that fixation type does not significantly affect fusion time or outcome (D Dennison, AY Shin, SL Moran, et al. Presented to the American Academy of Orthopaedic Surgeons, Chicago, Illinois, 2006; **Figure** 7). For significantly advanced arthritis involving the radiolunate joint or in patients with requirements for heavy lifting, total wrist arthrodesis is recommended. Before total wrist fusion, a short arm splint is tried. If the patient is unable to tolerate the splint, four-corner fusion may be attempted.

CONCLUSION

Long-standing scaphoid nonunion remains a difficult problem. It is hoped that earlier recognition and improvements in scaphoid fixation will decrease the incidence of this problem. For patients with established radiocarpal arthritis, some type of wrist salvage procedure should be considered to decrease pain and maintain motion.

REFERENCES

1. Fisk GR: An overview of injuries of the wrist. *Clin Orthop Rel Res* 1980:137-144.
2. Linscheid RL, Dobyns JH, Beckenbaugh RD, Cooney WP III, Wood MB: Instability patterns of the wrist. *J Hand Surg Am* 1983;8:682-686.
3. Weber ER: Biomechanical implications of scaphoid waist fractures. *Clin Orthop* 1980;149:83-89.
4. Smith DK, Cooney WP III, An KN, Linscheid RL, Chao EYS: The effects of simulated unstable scaphoid fractures on carpal motion. *J Hand Surg Am* 1989;14:283-291.
5. Smith DK, An KN, Cooney WP III, Linscheid RL, Chao EY: Effects of a scaphoid waist osteotomy on carpal kinematics. *J Orthop Res* 1989;7:590-598.
6. Viegas SF, Patterson RM, Hillman GR, Peterson PD, Crossley M, Foster R: Simulated scaphoid proximal pole fracture. *J Hand Surg Am* 1989;16:495-500.
7. Linscheid RL, Dobyns JH, Beabout JW, Bryan RS: Traumatic instability of the wrist: Diagnosis, classification, and pathomechanics. *J Bone Joint Surg Am* 1972;54:1612-1632.
8. Mack GR, Bosse MJ, Gelberman RH, Yu E: The natural history of scaphoid non-union. *J Bone Joint Surg Am* 1984;66:504-509.
9. Ruby LK, Stinson J, Belsky MR: The natural history of scaphoid non-union: A review of fifty-five cases. *J Bone Joint Surg Am* 1985;67:428-432.
10. Vender MI, Watson HK, Wiener BD, Black DM: Degenerative changes in symptomatic scaphoid nonunion. *J Hand Surg Am* 1987;12:514-519.
11. Moritomo H, Viegas SF, Elder KW, et al: Scaphoid nonunions: A three-dimensional analysis of patterns of deformity. *J Hand Surg Am* 2000;25:520-528.
12. Watson HK, Ballet FL: The SLAC wrist: Scapholunate advanced collapse pattern of degenerative arthritis. *J Hand Surg Am* 1984;9:358-365.
13. Watson HK, Weinzweig J, Zeppieri J: The natural progression of scaphoid instability. *Hand Clin* 1997;13:39-49.
14. Krakauer JD, Bishop AT, Cooney WP: Surgical treatment of scapholunate advanced collapse. *J Hand Surg Am* 1994;19:751-759.
15. Fisk GR: Carpal instability and the fractured scaphoid. *Ann R Coll Surg Engl* 1970;46:63-76.
16. Dickison JC, Shannon JG: Fractures of the carpal scaphoid in the Canadian Army. *Surg Gynecol Obstet* 1944;79:225-239.
17. London PS: The broken scaphoid bone: The case against pessimism. *J Bone Joint Surg Br* 1961;43:237-244.

18. London PS: Ununited fracture of the scaphoid bone, in *Proceedings of the Second Hand Club*. London, British Society for Surgery of the Hand, 1975, pp 1956-1967.

19. Mazet R, Hohl M: Conservative treatment of old fractures of the carpal scaphoid. *J Trauma* 1961;1:115-127.

20. Mazet R, Hohl M: Fractures of the carpal navicular: Analysis of 91 cases and review of the literature. *J Bone Joint Surg Am* 1963;45:82-112.

21. Martin MA: Carpal instability and scaphoid pseudarthrosis. *Rev Esp Cir Mano* 1995;50:25-32.

22. Kaneshiro SA, Faila JM, Tashman S: Scaphoid fracture displacement with forearm rotation in a short-arm thumb spica cast. *J Hand Surg Am* 1999;24:984-991.

23. Jupiter JB, Shin AY, Trumble TE, Fernandez DL: Traumatic and reconstructive problems of the scaphoid. *Instr Course Lect* 2001;50:105-122.

24. Bonnevialle P, Mansat M, Railhac JJ, Rongières M, Gay R: Radio-carpal and inter-carpal degenerative arthritis in sequelae of scaphoid injuries. *Ann Chir Main* 1987;6:89-97.

25. Milliez PY, Courandier JM, Thomine JM, Biga N: The natural history of scaphoid non-union: A review of fifty-two cases. *Ann Chir Main* 1987;6:195-202.

26. Kerluke I, McCabe SJ: Nonunion of the scaphoid: A critical analysis of recent natural history studies. *J Hand Surg Am* 1993;18:1-3.

27. Schuind F, Haetjens P, Van Innis F, Vander Marer C, Garcia-Elias M, Sennwald G: Prognostic factors in the treatment of carpal scaphoid nonunions. *J Hand Surg Am* 1999;24:761-776.

28. Shaw J, Jones WA: Factors affecting the outcome in 50 cases of scaphoid nonunion treated with Herbert screw fixation. *J Hand Surg Br* 1998;23:680-685.

29. Inoue G, Shionoya K, Kuwahata Y: Ununited proximal pole scaphoid fractures: Treatment with Herbert screw in 16 cases followed for 0.5-8 years. *Acta Orthop Scand* 1997;68:124-127.

30. Inoue G, Kuwahata Y: Repeat screw stabilization with bone grafting after failed Herbert screw fixation for acute scaphoid fractures and nonunions. *J Hand Surg Am* 1997;22: 413-418.

31. Buchler U, Nagy L: The issue of vascularity in fractures and nonunions of the scaphoid. *J Hand Surg Br* 1995;20:726-735.

32. Boyer MI, von Schroeder HP, Axelrod TS: Scaphoid nonunion with avascular necrosis of the proximal pole: Treatment with a vascularized bone graft from the dorsum of the distal radius. *J Hand Surg Br* 1998;23:686-690.

33. Straw RG, Davis TR, Dias JJ: Scaphoid nonunion: Treatment with a pedicled vascularized bone graft based on the 1,2 intercompartmental supraretinacular branch of the radial artery. *J Hand Surg Br* 2002;27:413-416.

34. Perlik PC, Guilford WB: Magnetic resonance imaging to assess vascularity of scaphoid non-unions. *J Hand Surg Am* 1991;16:479-484.

35. Morgan WJ, Breen TF, Coumas JM, Schulz LA: Role of magnetic resonance imaging in assessing factors affecting healing in scaphoid nonunions. *Clin Orthop* 1997;336:240-246.

36. Downing ND, Oni JA, Davis TR, Vu TQ, Dawson JS, Martel AL: The relationship between proximal pole blood flow and the subjective assessment of increased density of the proximal pole in acute scaphoid fractures. *J Hand Surg Am* 2002;27:402-408.

37. Gunal I, Ozcelik A, Gokturk E, Ada, S, Demirtas M: Correlation of magnetic resonance imaging and intra-operative punctate bleeding to assess the casularity of scaphoid union. *Arch Orthop Trauma Surg* 1999;119:285-287.

38. Cerezal L, Abascal F, Canga A, Farcia-Valtuille R, Bustamante M, Pinal F: Utility of gadolinium-enhanced MR in the evaluation of the vascularity of scaphoid nonunions. *Am J Roentgenol* 2000;174:141-149.

39. Nakamura T, Cooney WP III, Lui WH, et al: Radial styloidectomy: A biomechanical study on stability of the wrist joint. *J Hand Surg Am* 2001;26:85-93.

40. Siegel DB, Gelberman RH: Radial styloidectomy: An anatomical study with special reference to radiocarpal intracapsular ligamentous morphology. *J Hand Surg Am* 1991;16:40-44.

41. Barnard L, Stubbins SG: Styloidectomy of the radius in the surgical treatment of non-union of the carpal navicular. *J Bone Joint Surg Am* 1948;30:98-102.

42. Brunelli GA, Brunelli GR: A personal technique for treatment of scaphoid non-union. *J Hand Surg Br* 1991;16:148-152.

43. Pennsylvania Orthopedic Society SRC: Evaluation of treatment for non-union of the carpal navicular. *J Bone Joint Surg Am* 1962;44:169-174.

44. Cooney WP III, Dobyns JH, Linscheid RL: Nonunion of the scaphoid: Analysis of the results from bone grafting. *J Hand Surg Am* 1980;5:343-354.

45. Sprague B, Justis EJ: Nonunion of the carpal navicular: Modes of treatment. *Arch Surg* 1974;108:692-697.

46. Haussman P: Long-term results after silicone prosthesis replacement of the proximal pole of the scaphoid bone in advanced scaphoid nonunion. *J Hand Surg Br* 2002;27:417-423.

47. Alexander AH, Turner MA, Alexander CE, Lichtman DW: Lunate silicone replacement arthroplasty in Kienböck's disease: A long-term follow-up. *J Hand Surg Am* 1990;15:401-407.

48. Egloff DV, Varadi G, Narakas A, Simonetta C, Cantero C: Silastic implants of the scaphoid and lunate: A long term clinical study with a mean follow-up of 13 years. *J Hand Surg Br* 1993;18:687-692.

49. Carter PR, Benton LJ, Dysert PA: Silicone rubber carpal implants: A study of the incidence of late osseous complications. *J Hand Surg Am* 1986;11:639-644.

50. Gordon M, Bullough PG: Synovial and osseous inflammation in failed silicone-rubber prostheses: A report of six cases. *J Bone Joint Surg Am* 1982;64:574-580.

51. Peimer CA, Medige J, Eckert BS, Wright JR, Howard CS: Reactive synovitis after silicone arthroplasty. *J Hand Surg Am* 1986;11:624-638.

52. Rosenthal DI, Rosenberg AE, Schiller AL, Smith RJ: Destructive arthritis due to silicone: A foreign body reaction. *Radiology* 1983;149:69-72.

53. Smith DJ, Sazy JA, Crissman JD, Niu Z-T, Robson MC, Heggers JP: Immunogenic potential of carpal implants. *J Surg Res* 1990;48:132-120.

54. Smith RJ, Atkinson RE, Jupiter JB: Silicone synovitis of the wrist. *J Hand Surg Am* 1985;10:47-60.

55. Wickham MG, Rudolph R, Abraham JL: Silicone identification in prosthesis-associated fibrous capsule. *Science* 1978;199:437-439.

56. Vinnars B, Adamsson L, af Ekenstam F, Wadin K, Gerdin B: Patient-rating of long term results of silicone implant arthroplasty of the scaphoid. *Scand J Plast Reconstr Surg* 2002;36:39-45.

57. Weinstein LP, Berger RA: Analgesic benefit, functional outcome, and patient satisfaction after partial wrist denervation. *J Hand Surg Am* 2002;27:833-839.

58. Dellon A, Mackinnon S, Daneshvar A: Terminal branch of the anterior interosseous nerve as a source of wrist pain. *J Hand Surg Br* 1984;9:316-322.

59. Bentzon PGK, Madsen AR: Surgical therapy of pseudarthrosis following fractures of carpal scaphoid bone. *Nord Med* 1944;21:524.

60. Rasmussen KB: Bentzon's operation for pseudarthrosis of the scaphoid bone (abstract). *J Bone Joint Surg Br* 1963;45:621.

61. Agner O: Treatment of ununited fractures of the carpal scaphoid by Bentzon's operation. *Acta Orthop Scand* 1963;33:56-65.

62. Boeckstyns MEH, Busch P: Surgical treatment of scaphoid pseudarthrosis: Evaluation of the results after soft tissue arthroplasty and inlay bone grafting. *J Hand Surg Am* 1984;9:378-382.

63. Boeckstyns MEH, Kajäer L, Busch P, Holst-Nielsen F: Soft tissue interposition arthroplasty for scaphoid nonunion. *J Hand Surg Am* 1985;10:109-114.

64. Malerich MM, Clifford J, Eaton B, Eaton R, Littler J: Distal scaphoid resection arthroplasty for the treatment of degenerative arthritis secondary to scaphoid nonunion. *J Hand Surg Am* 1999;24:1196-1205.

65. Ruch DS, Chang DS, Poehling GG: The arthroscopic treatment of avascular necrosis of the proximal pole following scaphoid nonunion. *Arthroscopy* 1998;14:747-752.

66. Ruch DS, Chang DS, Yang B: Arthroscopic evaluation and treatment of scaphoid nonunion. *Hand Clin* 2001;17:655-662.

67. Soejima O, Iida H, Hanamura T, Naito M: Resection of the distal pole of the scaphoid for scaphoid nonunion with radioscaphoid and intercarpal arthritis. *J Hand Surg Am* 2003;28:591-596.

68. Hill NA: Fractures and dislocations of the carpus. *Orthop Clin North Am* 1970;1:275.

69. Crabbe WA: Excision of the proximal row of the carpus. *J Bone Joint Surg Br* 1964;46:708-711.

70. Inglis AE, Jones EC: Proximal-row carpectomy for diseases of the proximal row. *J Bone Joint Surg Am* 1977;59:460-463.

71. Jorgensen TM, Andresen JH, Thommesen P, Hansen HH: Scanning and radiology of the carpal scaphoid bone. *Acta Orthop Scand* 1979;50:663-665.

72. Arcalis A, Pedemonte J: Proximal row carpectomy for advanced nonunion of the scaphoid. *Rev Orthop Trauma* 1998;42:39-41.

73. Jebson PJ, Hayes E, Engber WD: Proximal row carpectomy: A minimum 10-year follow-up study. *J Hand Surg* 2003;28:561-569.

74. DiDonna M, Kiefhaber T, Stern PJ: Proximal row carpectomy: Study with a minimum of ten years of follow-up. *J Bone Joint Surg Am* 2004;86:2359-2365.

75. Sutro CJ: Treatment of nonunion of the carpal navicular bone. *Surgery* 1946;20:536.

76. Helfet AJ: A new operation for ununited fracture of the scaphoid (abstract). *J Bone Joint Surg Br* 1952;34:329.

77. Gordon LH, King D: Partial wrist arthrodesis for old ununited fractures of the carpal navicular. *Am J Surg* 1961;102:460-464.

78. Graner O, Lopes E, Costa-Carvalho B, Atlas S: Arthrodesis of the carpal bones in the treatment of Kienböck's disease, painful un-united fractures of the navicular and lunate bones with avascular necrosis, and old fracture-dislocations of carpal bones. *J Bone Joint Surg Am* 1966;48:767-774.

79. Mack GR, Lichtman DM: Scaphoid nonunion, in Lichtman DM (ed): *The Wrist and Its Disorders*, Philadelphia, PA, WB Saunders, 1988, pp 293-328.

80. Viegas SF, Patterson RM, Peterson PD, Crossley M, Foster R: The silicone scaphoid: A biomechanical study. *J Hand Surg Am* 1991;16:91-97.

81. Toby EB, Glisson RR, Seaber AV, Urbaniak JR: Prosthetic silicone scaphoid strains: Effects of intercarpal fusions. *J Hand Surg Am* 1991;16:469-473.

82. Eaton RG, Akelman E, Eaton BH: Fascial implant arthroplasty for treatment of radioscaphoid degenerative disease. *J Hand Surg Am* 1989;14:766-774.

83. Watson H, Ryu J: Evolution of arthritis of the wrist. *Clin Orthop* 1986;202:57-67.

84. Ashmead D IV, Watson HK, Damon C, Herber S, Paly W: Scapholunate advanced collapse wrist salvage. *J Hand Surg Am* 1994;19:741-750.

85. Tomaino MM, Miller R, Cole I, Burton RI: Scapholunate advanced collapse wrist: Proximal row carpectomy or limited wrist arthrodesis with scaphoid excision? *J Hand Surg Am* 1994;19:134-142.

86. Wyrick J, Stern P, Kiefhaber T: Motion-preserving procedures in the treatment of scapholunate advanced collapse wrist: Proximal row carpectomy versus four-corner arthrodesis. *J Hand Surg Am* 1995;20:965-970.

87. Cohen MS, Kozin SH: Degenerative arthritis of the wrist: Proximal row carpectomy versus scaphoid excision and four-corner arthrodesis. *J Hand Surg Am* 2001;26:94-104.

88. Vance M, Hernandez J, DiDonna M, Stern P: Complications and outcome of four-corner arthrodesis: Circular plate fixation versus traditional techniques. *J Hand Surg Am* 2005;30:1122-1127.

89. Viegas SF, Patterson RM, Peterson PD, et al: Evaluation of the biomechanical efficacy of limited intercarpal fusions for the treatment of scapho-lunate dissociations. *J Hand Surg Am* 1990;15:120-128.

90. Kirschenbaum D, Schneider L, Kirkpatrick W, Adams D, Cody R: Scaphoid excision and capitolunate arthrodesis for radioscaphoid arthritis. *J Hand Surg Am* 1993;18:780-785.

91. Kadji O, Duteille F, Dautel G, Merle M: Four bone versus capito-lunate limited carpal fusion: Report of 40 cases. *Chir Main* 2002;21:5-12.

92. Calandruccio JH, Gelberman R, Duncan SF, Goldfarb CA, Pae R, Gramig W: Capitolunate arthrodesis with scaphoid and triquetrum excision. *J Hand Surg Am* 2000;25:824-832.

93. Imbriglia JE, Broudy A, Hagberg W, McKernan D: Proximal row carpectomy: Clinical evaluation. *J Hand Surg Am* 1990;15:426-430.

94. Salomon G, Eaton R: Proximal row carpectomy with partial capitate resection. *J Hand Surg Am* 1996;21:2-8.

95. Murphy D, Khoury G, Imbriglia JE, Adams BD: Comparison of arthroplasty and arthrodesis for rheumatoid wrist. *J Hand Surg Am* 2003;28:570-576.

96. Adams BD, Grosland N, Murphy D, McCullough M: Impact of impaired wrist motion on hand and upper-extremity performance. *J Hand Surg Am* 2003;28:898-903.

97. Hastings H II, Weiss AP, Quenzer DE, Wiedeman G, Hanington K, Strickland JW: Arthrodesis of the wrist for post-traumatic disorders. *J Bone Joint Surg* 1996;78:897-902.

INDEX